Life after
Cancer

Life after Cancer:

Coping with a Cancer Verdict

Eliezer Benaroya

iUniverse, Inc.
New York   Bloomington

Life After Cancer:
Coping with a Cancer Verdict

iUniverse books may be ordered through booksellers or by contacting:

iUniverse
1663 Liberty Drive
Bloomington, IN 47403
www.iuniverse.com
1-800-Authors (1-800-288-4677)

ISBN: 978-0-595-47759-3 (pbk)
ISBN: 978-0-595-71355-4 (cloth)
ISBN: 978-1-4401-0891-4 (ebk)

Printed in the United States of America

iUniverse rev. 02/09/2009

This book is written in loving memory of my father ABRAHAM BENAROYA who taught me the values of hard work, optimism, patios, perseverance and courage. And to my mother ALEGRA EFTIMIA BENAROYA who gave me unconditional love throughout my life in spite of my many shortcomings, and inserted in me the value and the power of family.

Contents

Preface

I wrote this book for all cancer patients who are in the same situation I was when I was first diagnosed with cancer. The feeling of not knowing what the future holds can be very scary, and it helps to learn from others who have gone down a similar path. The battle against cancer is worthwhile: even if it seems at first glance like the end of the world, not only can you prolong your life, but you can maintain a reasonable quality of it. I want to deliver a message of hope, to reassure you there can be a good life waiting for you after cancer.

Two years have passed since I was first diagnosed with colon cancer. I've gone through three surgeries, six months of chemotherapy, and many months of recovery. Today I consider myself very lucky to be alive. I'm enjoying a life filled with traveling, adventure, discovery, family, and love. Aside from a few limitations, I can still experience everything I did before being diagnosed with cancer—and maybe even more.

Now when flying, I take an extra carry-on containing my medical supplies (not luggage I want to lose), and at times I experience skin irritation in high-humidity environments, but no life is perfect, as everyone has his or her "baggage." I can still enjoy many activities such as hiking, running, swimming, and almost anything else I feel like doing. Sometimes I take extra precautions specific to my situation, such as waiting for convenient hours to eat or staying away from certain foods to avoid an overactive ostomy. If I'd never been diagnosed with cancer, I probably would still be working at the deli, feeling overstressed and not experiencing nearly as many things as I am today.

Of course, I need to be vigilant and be tested every six months to make sure the cancer hasn't come back. But if I didn't have to monitor my cancer, I might wait years before going to a doctor, which might allow some other disease or condition to go undetected.

I also want to make sure you know your allies in the battle against cancer. The medical professionals are there to help, so use them. In turn, I would recommend to medical professionals that they try to invest more time in knowing each individual patient. If doctors would listen to their patients' thoughts and fears, they could better treat ailments and help their patients feel more comfortable with what the doctors are doing.

There is much more to healing than just its physical aspects, as emotional and spiritual factors also play a huge role. A patient's attitude toward any illness can make a big difference in his or her recovery. Changing the way you look at things can completely change how you recover. A positive outlook is an important aspect of one's ability to recover from a serious injury or illness. Throughout my illness, I had many ups and downs, but I never lost hope I could get beyond it.

My hope is that in the not-so-distant future, cancer will become a better understood disease with well-established treatments. As my small part to help in this effort, a portion of the proceeds from this book will be donated to cancer research.

1
The Whole Nine Miles

It was a few days before my fifty-sixth birthday, a routine Saturday on which my friend Motty and I were going jogging. Almost every weekend Motty and I would jog around the beautiful Lake Chabot in Castro Valley, California, just a few miles away from my home. Motty is a longtime friend who has been instrumental in igniting in me the enthusiasm for running long distances.

A few years back at our first run around Lake Chabot together (Motty had already been a frequent runner there for many years), he told me the distance around the lake was about four or five miles, which was only a little longer than what I was used to running. Only after we completed the run did he announce the true distance: nine miles. I was very surprised I'd been able to complete it as it was something I probably wouldn't even have attempted had I known. It was a real thrill for me to be able to run the nine miles around the lake at the age of fifty-six—in fact, I felt on top of the world. I felt so good during the run that I began contemplating running a marathon before I got too old. At 26.2 miles, a marathon would be just about three times the distance of our weekend run. As Motty had already run several marathons himself, he strongly encouraged this idea.

On this particular day, the run was going very well and we were about to finish our route. It generally took us a little under an hour and a half to complete the run, and today was no different. Then we both headed to the water fountain to replace all the fluids we'd lost.

Once rehydrated, we walked to the stretching area where we spent a few minutes before returning to the car that was parked about half a mile away. Motty released the car key from his shoelace and opened the door to his twenty-year-old Toyota Supra. Motty is very proud of his Supra and often says, "It has over two hundred thousand miles and still runs like it's new." As he was getting the car open, I used the time to stretch a bit more.

But then I stood up and suddenly felt dizzy. I passed out for a few seconds, falling on the top of the car. It took a few minutes for me to get in the car, but Motty hardly noticed anything. I didn't mention anything to him during our ride home, but I was baffled as to what had just happened to me.

For some time now I had been feeling dizzy during the run, and I had no explanation for it. I was also falling asleep much more than usual, but I didn't think twice about it. About four years prior I'd had a complete physical, or so I thought, and my doctor was so happy with the results that he told me I should frame them because "this is as good as it gets."

It took twenty minutes for us to arrive at my house. I said good-bye to Motty and headed straight for the door. Shoshi, my beautiful wife of thirty-one years, opened the door with a big welcoming smile and a good-morning kiss. As Motty and I started our runs early in the morning, she was usually still asleep when I left the house.

When we sat down for breakfast together, I told her what happened after the run. She looked worried, and although I didn't think it was anything serious, I agreed to consult our physician about it.

On Monday morning I called my physician's office to make an appointment, but the earliest opening was two months away. I'm not a hypochondriac—quite the opposite in fact, as I'm the first person to dismiss pain or find explanations for it that doesn't include illness. I also rarely take medications or visit doctors. But this time was different, as I was worried that something was seriously wrong with me. For some time I'd been complaining to my family about a strange sensation I often felt in my stomach. The best way to describe it would be like a sudden drop in my gut, the way you feel on a rollercoaster ride, so I insisted on being seen that day. The secretary informed me that my physician, Dr. S, was not available, but I could come in to see his partner Dr. T later that afternoon. I immediately agreed and arrived a few hours later.

Dr. T seemed like a very nice man. He spoke with a Russian accent and looked to be about fifty. He had a very serious look on his face as he asked me about my symptoms. I described my experience that weekend, and then he examined me. He didn't notice anything unusual during his examination, but he saw that I had a very short record of office visits. He suggested I wear a heart monitor for twenty-four hours to test if my heart was experiencing any problems under different stress levels. I agreed and returned the next day to get the monitor hooked up.

2
Playing Detective

As a good detective would do, Dr. T tried to isolate the guilty organ from several suspects through a process of elimination. Suspect number one was my heart, with the monitor acting as a polygraph to see if it was really behaving the way it appeared during the visit. I wore the monitor for the next twenty-four hours everywhere I went.

Going to work with it was very embarrassing. I wore my colored long-sleeve shirt, leaving it untucked so no one would see the monitor, but this was very unusual for me as at work, I always wore a tucked-in white polo shirt. At the time my wife and I owned a deli in the marina of Alameda, and we had a very regular clientele. Everybody noticed I was dressed differently, but I continued to make up explanations for my change in attire.

In the evening when I got home, Motty called to see if I wanted to go for a walk. I hesitated for a minute because I didn't want him to know that I had a heart monitor. However, in the end I decided to join him in order to test the monitor at a different activity level. Once again, I hid the monitor under my untucked shirt, and we walked for about four miles through the hills of Palomares.

On Thursday morning I went back to the doctor's office so he could take the readings off the monitor. Dr. T asked how I felt, and I said I was fine; the nurse disconnected the electrodes, and I was released. I was asked to call back in two days to get the results.

After a very long forty-eight hours where every possible scenario raced through my mind from a possible heart attack to a blood circulation problem, I called the office and found out my heart was fine. Once the first organ was found innocent, Dr. T had to go back in search of new clues. The next step was to order blood and stool tests.

I came to the office the next morning to pick up the test orders, and then I went down the hall to the lab where some of my blood was taken. For the stool test I was given a kit to take home so I could provide three samples taken at different times. I did the samples as requested, not expecting to hear anything alarming. After all, only a few years had passed since my last physical whose results had been practically perfect. In addition, I'd never noticed any unusual bleeding, such as blood in my stool.

However, three days later when I got home from work, I found a disturbing message on the answering machine: "This is Dr. S's office calling for Eliezer. We received your test results. Please contact our office ASAP." I froze for a minute. After my heart had been cleared, I'd convinced myself that it was all a false alarm, but now my thoughts of relief changed again to worries and confusion. I then dialed the office number, but it was around 5:30 p.m. on Friday and the office was already closed. I wouldn't be able to call back until Monday morning, so my family and I had a very long weekend.

Come Monday morning, I woke up at 5:00 a.m. to go to work. The deli was open from 7:00 a.m. to 5:00 p.m., but employees started coming in at 6:00 a.m. to prepare for the day. Shoshi and I had a system in which I would go in early to open, with her coming in later and staying to close. As usual, she arrived around 10:00 a.m., and I immediately went into my office to call the doctor regarding Friday's message. It had been bothering me since then, as I'd thought of a million different things that could be wrong with me.

However, at first I was relieved as Dr. T told me the reason for the Friday call; it was worrisome, but not as bad as what I'd built it up to be in my head. He told me I was anemic, meaning I was losing blood. He asked me to come into the office to see him, so I scheduled an appointment for later that afternoon.

I was a bit anxious, as if they needed me to come in that same day, maybe it was more serious than I'd originally thought. I arrived thirty minutes early to my appointment, identified myself at the window, and then waited to be called in. Dr. T greeted me with a handshake and asked me to have a seat. He then told me I was losing blood from somewhere, most likely from my colon either from colon cancer or another colon injury. Another possibility was an ulcer.

His tone of voice was very calm and although the word *cancer* was mentioned, I wasn't alarmed as mentally I dismissed it as only a theoretical possibility. He recommended having a colonoscopy performed to see if we could convict the second suspect, my colon. Dr. T gave me information about the gastrointestinal (GI) doctor they generally referred patients to but gave me the option to choose my own doctor.

The name he mentioned was familiar to me, as my wife and I had met him years ago. When we were new immigrants to this country and completely broke, we wanted to send our two boys to camp one summer. The camp was subsidized for low-income families, but the camp administration required a clear bill of health before accepting the children. At the time we couldn't afford health insurance, and a doctor's visit would be too costly. I'd told Shoshi we should just forget the whole thing, as it was too embarrassing, but my wife was more persistent. Shoshi is not a person who gives up easily, so she asked the rabbi at our temple for some help. In no time, our rabbi found us a doctor who would perform the physical for our children free of charge.

This was the same person Dr. T was now mentioning to me, so the doctor who helped my children twenty years ago was now going to perform my colonoscopy. We were very thankful when he'd helped us in the past, and I was happy to go to someone familiar to me as I felt I was in good hands. I left Dr. T's office and walked down one floor to make an appointment for my colonoscopy.

3
The Discovery

The day of the exam, I arrived at the clinic with my son Avi and my daughter Orit. I'd spent most of the previous night in the bathroom cleaning out my colon with the help of a nasty beverage called Fleet. After I checked in at the clinic, I was led to a bed, asked to remove all my clothes, and given a gown to put on. They handed me some paperwork to fill out, and I started reading about all the possible side effects and risks associated with the procedure I was about to have done. They were routine documents designed to release everyone involved from any liability, but while reading about these risks, I began to get cold feet about the whole thing. It was the first time in my life I'd felt this way, lying in a clinic bed about to have what I thought to be some kind of surgery.

The curtain moved and I saw in front of me the familiar face of the doctor who'd helped my children years ago. He said, "You're next—are you ready?" I wasn't ready. "Doctor, do I really need this procedure?" I asked. He answered me in an angry voice, "You are over fifty, aren't you? Of course you need it!" He left without leaving me time to comment. I felt very uneasy. He had a reputation as a good GI doctor, but the way he talked to me wasn't exactly what I'd expected from him.

The nurse came and started an intravenous (IV) line, then rolled the bed to the room where the procedure would take place. As I was being sedated through the IV, two nurses were preparing the equipment, and I remember them placing the monitor to my left. When the doctor walked in, he tried to engage me in small talk about our temple to help me relax. He'd served as president of our temple a few years back but was no longer an active member. He then asked me to turn to the left, which placed my face directly in front of the monitor. I felt like I was watching some interesting science movie, but it was the inside of my body I was actually seeing.

An instrument was inserted through my rectum and started traveling through my colon. I could see inside of my colon when the probe was moving slowly, inch by inch. It was not very painful, and it was only about fifteen minutes until I heard the doctor's voice saying, "Here is the source of your bleeding." "What is it?" I asked. "It's a tumor," he uttered very calmly. "Is it malignant?" "Yes, and it has to come out." Through the monitor I could see him cutting two pieces of what I assumed was my tumor to send to the lab, and then I saw the instrument coming out. Suddenly, it was over.

At that point I felt relieved the colonoscopy hadn't been as painful as I'd feared. As I was rolled out of the room, I noticed quite a few people were waiting for the same procedure.

The doctor rushed to write the report, which he then handed to me. It included a colorful photo of my tumor. He told me to take the report to my physician, Dr. S, and to begin looking for a surgeon right away. "How long has the tumor been there?" I asked. "At least five years," he responded.

My mind went completely blank. I couldn't comprehend that I

was being informed of my cancer in such a cold voice. I felt numb and not really sure what needed to be done next, or by whom. Physically I felt very good and couldn't grasp that I'd just been diagnosed with cancer. The people I knew who had cancer did not look good, but my image in the mirror didn't indicate anything was wrong.

The nurse came in and asked me to get dressed, and then she brought me a wheelchair. My son Avi was pushing my wheelchair through the corridor leading to the parking lot. The nurse walked with us, holding my hand tightly the whole way. She was very empathetic, and I could see in her face that she wasn't very happy with the way the doctor had broken the news to me.

As Avi drove me home, I told him the news. As soon as I got home, the phone rang. It was Shoshi, who had probably been trying to call for some time waiting to hear the results of the colonoscopy. "Well, what happened?" she asked. "Nothing," I said. "The doctor said I have a tumor that has to come out." I passed the phone to Avi, who gave her the details. I wasn't in any mood to talk on the phone, especially about what had just happened. It was too fresh in my mind, and I had to let the news settle.

4
The Battle Begins

My colonoscopy was performed on August 17, 2004, and Dr. A hadn't even needed to wait for the biopsy report to know the tumor was malignant. I quickly realized that before I could make any decisions, I needed to get educated on the subject. I began to research the disease, and all possible cures. I found through my research the symptoms of colon cancer are:

- A change in bowel habits
- Blood in the stool
- Diarrhea/constipation
- Narrower than usual stool
- Abdominal pain
- Weight loss
- Vomiting

Of all these symptoms, the only one I'd experienced was blood in my stool, and it wasn't even visible to the naked eye.

On August 18th, the day after my colonoscopy, the biopsy report confirmed I had an adenocarcinoma of the ascending colon, a.k.a colon cancer. The next step was to assemble the troops for the fight. Everyone in my family rolled up his or her sleeves and went to work. My daughter helped substitute for my wife and me at the deli when we had to be absent. We all began our research, buying books and spending many hours on the Internet with the help of Google, just gathering as much information as we could to help us understand this disease.

Although I wanted to be true to my philosophy regarding minimal intervention, I very quickly realized doing nothing was not a good option. Aside from the high risk of the cancer spreading, I couldn't keep losing blood.

On August 19th I was back in Dr. S's office. The colonoscopy and biopsy reports were already on his desk. He immediately ordered X-rays to be taken the same day and recommended a surgeon in the local hospital who could remove the tumor. I walked over to the adjacent building for my X-ray, and after I was done, I went to schedule an appointment with the surgeon. Her earliest opening was for the 21st, so I took it. Then I went back to Radiology to check on the X-ray results. They were ready, but I had to take them back to Dr. S to get my report.

As I walked back to Dr. S's office, I was happy that at least everything was close by so I didn't have to drive around like a madman. The X-ray showed no abnormalities, so the next test Dr. S ordered was a computed tomography (CT) scan to see if the cancer had spread to any other organs. He told me the surgeon would need the report, so I scheduled the scan for the next day.

On August 20th, the CT scan was performed. It did not show any spread of the cancer, and I was relieved. Meanwhile through his Internet search, my son Yaniv had found a surgeon, Dr. W., at Stanford Hospital. Yaniv lives in Hawaii, and he had just flown in to join us for the appointment with the surgeon Dr. S recommended. However, Yaniv thought Dr. W. would be a good consultant because of his extensive experience, including working at UCSF for several years before moving to Stanford.

The next day, August 21st, was my appointment with the surgeon Dr. S had referred me to. Yaniv and Shoshi were with me as we entered the office. There was only one patient ahead of us, so we sat down and immediately engaged in conversation with her. It turned out she was very happy to be a patient of the surgeon's, and she didn't stop praising the surgeon until she was finally called in.

When our turn came, we went into the room and I sat down on the bed in its center. There was a big picture of a colon hanging on the wall, and I examined it very carefully. This was the first time I'd seen a diagram of the human colon, and it was very different from what I'd envisioned.

The doctor came in and began explaining my situation. I had a sizable tumor in my ascending colon, which could be removed through surgery. Normal recovery would take about one week, and she didn't foresee any complications. Of course there were no guarantees, as all surgeries carry a risk, but she performed this surgery weekly and made it seem like no big deal. According to her, my cancer was very common in men and women over fifty, and if detected early enough, a full recovery was expected. To me it was a much bigger deal, but we scheduled the surgery for the following week because she made sure to remind us that time was of the essence.

We were about to leave when Yaniv asked her if she knew Dr. W from Stanford Hospital. She did know him, and she spoke highly of him. She mentioned that she usually referred her complicated cases to him, but my case was very simple and she would have no problem with it. We thanked her and proceeded to the window to make an appointment for the surgery.

On the way home we discussed what she had said about Dr. W, and all agreed that if Dr. W was the one who performed the complicated surgeries, he would definitely be good for me. Without even realizing it, she'd talked us out of surgery with her and sold us on Dr. W. We got home and Yaniv immediately scheduled an appointment with Dr. W.

Then Yaniv called his business partner's father for some advice. The father was a retired podiatrist, and although he wasn't very familiar with my condition, he knew a thing or two about the medical system. He gave us some very good advice: keep all medical records in one binder and take them to every appointment we had. A lot of time can be wasted searching for and sending records back and forth, but this way my entire medical history would be ready for every doctor to see. From that day on, I asked for copies of every single test I had. This advice turned out to be very helpful, and it was a huge asset in my battle against cancer.

5
Choices and Decisions

My appointment with Dr. W was on Tuesday, August 24th. We had a long list of questions written down from a family brainstorming session the night before. We didn't want to forget anything during the appointment, as we had done in the past.

Some of our questions were:

- How long is the surgery?
- What is the healing time after surgery?
- Will there be a change in functionality after surgery?
- When do we need to see an oncologist?
- Are there any foods that I should avoid?
- Any foods I should focus on?
- How about exercise—should it be limited before surgery or increased?
- Is colon cancer surgery your specialty?

We knew that many more questions would come up during the

appointment, but we wanted to have a list prepared with everything we could think of.

The drive from our house to Stanford Hospital took about an hour, and during the entire ride, there was a tense silence in the car. I was fantasizing that Dr. W would examine me and tell me that it was all a big mistake, that I was perfectly healthy. Obviously that's not what happened.

When my name was called, I walked down a long corridor to the nurse's station where I had my blood pressure, weight, and temperature taken. They then escorted me to a room down the hall to wait for Dr. W.

After about twenty minutes, five doctors walked in. One of them introduced the group as medical students, shook our hands, and asked a few questions while recording the answers. Then he asked if it would be okay to perform a rectal exam. After he was done, they all left the room, announcing they would be back with Dr. W shortly. As soon as the door closed, I suddenly realized that my body would be used for the benefit of new doctors, and I actually felt good about being able to contribute to the training of the next generation of health care professionals.

Stanford University is adjacent to Stanford Hospital, which is known for being a teaching hospital. Each patient must give consent to allow the students to be involved in the medical process, including the actual surgery. I knew the university was located next to the hospital, but the intense involvement of the students in all medical activities in the hospital was a surprise to me. However, I thought it was a worthwhile price to pay for having the best treatment possible.

A few minutes after the five students left, Dr. W came into my room with a large entourage of the same medical students and some new faces of resident doctors behind him. He shook our hands and sat down. He gave us detailed descriptions of my condition with the aid of a colon he drew on a piece of paper. According to Dr. W, surgery was my best option. When I asked about the risks, he told me the odds of my being killed in a car accident on my way home were much greater than dying from complications during surgery. Monday was the only time he had available because Tuesday morning he was flying to Hawaii to give several lectures.

He gave us a few minutes alone to discuss our available options. I felt very comfortable with Dr. W: he was not only very well qualified, but friendly and easy to talk to. I was somewhat concerned that he was leaving for a week after the surgery and wouldn't be around to oversee my recovery, but he assured us Dr. S, the other surgeon in the department, would be taking care of me. I felt comfortable with this, and Yaniv and Shoshi both agreed, so we decided to cancel the appointment we had scheduled with the other surgeon and go with Dr. W instead.

At that point, the nurse coordinator came in to ask us what we'd decided, and we informed her that we wanted to schedule the surgery with Dr. W. She began the process immediately. I was given a stack of forms to fill out, and then taken to the last window at the end of the corridor to schedule the surgery time. Before we left, the nurse coordinator prepped me on what I would feel after coming out of the operating room, as she wanted to make sure I didn't have any unrealistic expectations. According to her, I would feel like I had just been run over by a truck.

She also recommended buying a cheap pair of slippers for my hospital stay that could be disposed of as soon as I was discharged, because as hospitals are not very clean environments, she advised against bringing anything home from there. Then she mentioned they would insert a tube through my nose to extract fluids from my stomach. She told me that if everything went well, they would take this tube out before I woke up, but about 50 percent of the time it needed to stay in for a few days longer. If that were my situation, they would then have to take it out while I was awake, and it could be very uncomfortable. "I hope you will be able to avoid that," she said. Finally she promised to come visit me after surgery, and although I guessed it was just a nice gesture, it was still good to hear.

On the day following my visit with Dr. W, I received many phone calls from concerned family members and friends from the United States, Israel, and Greece. One of these calls was from my wife's niece Nitza, who gave us the phone number of her co-worker's brother, a GI doctor in Indianapolis, Indiana. She thought he might be able to give us some advice, so after hesitating for two days, I decided to give Dr. H a call. I didn't expect much from that conversation—he didn't know me, and doctors tend to have very busy schedules. At the most I expected a brief explanation of my problem possibly followed by some comforting remarks.

However, Dr. H spent more than half an hour helping me understand that I'd made the right choice to have the surgery. As someone who had never before confronted a major medical challenge, having a surgery was a momentous decision, and being reassured I'd made the right one was very helpful. From that day on, Dr. H took a personal interest in my progress, and we became very good friends. We would talk and e-mail weekly; I also always faxed him my test results, and he would call me back with explanations confirming what my doctors were telling me. This gave me confidence I was doing the right thing, especially as all of this was coming from an educated, unbiased third party. It was very helpful for me to have this outside perspective because most of my knowledge of what was going on was from what others were telling me. When his information matched the doctors' information, it was very comforting. I felt very lucky as well as grateful to have Dr. H to guide me through this lengthy process of surgery and recovery. To this day I have not met Dr. H or his wife, but a very good friendship has developed between our families.

The next step I had to take immediately was to train my wife Shoshi on all our financial matters. Up to that point I was the one responsible for paying the bills, and it was important to ensure continuity through my recovery. She also needed to know about all the bank accounts, insurance policies, and all the other financial matters with which she had not been involved prior to my diagnosis. I also shared all this information with my children so they would be able to help my wife in the event I didn't make it through surgery or had to endure a prolonged hospital stay.

At the meeting with Dr. W, he discussed the options I had for cleaning up my system before surgery, similar to what I'd done before my colonoscopy. The first option was Fleet, which comes in a four-ounce bottle and is to be taken in two doses, diluted with a little bit of water. The second option was GoLYTELY, which is an entire gallon of fluid that must be consumed. Neither of these options was appealing at all, and I dreaded the thought of drinking either of these beverages. The surgery itself was enough to bear.

Therefore, when Dr. W mentioned an experiment he was conducting with other doctors on the need for using this kind of medication, I listened closely. Although it made it less messy for the surgeon, he didn't think it was necessary to clean up the system prior to surgery. Dr. W asked if I'd be willing to participate in his research, which would include two groups of patients: half would use the medication to clean their systems while the other half would not. Both groups would be followed to determine if those using one method fared better than the other. Computers would randomly determine which group I would be placed in, but I was very eager to participate. Without participating, I would have to take the medication for sure; this way I had a 50/50 chance of avoiding it. However, to my disappointment, the computer placed me in the group required to take the medication.

6
The First Surgery

Yaniv and I arrived at the hospital early in the morning on August 27th for some final tests. Because I'd been squeezed into the surgeon's schedule at the last minute, the anesthesiologist wouldn't have time to see me until the day of surgery. However, I met with a nurse who took some blood while someone else performed an electrocardiogram to make sure my heart could handle the surgery. The nurse informed me that my heart looked good. On the way home, I told Yaniv I felt good about the decision to have the surgery done at Stanford Hospital as they seemed very professional and sincere.

In the next few days leading to my surgery, I ran three to four miles every day as I thought it would help my recovery if I was in good shape. My thoughts were on the day after surgery when I had a role to play in the recovery stage. I wasn't so worried about the surgery itself, as I had full confidence in my surgeon, and at that point there was nothing I could do to help.

The day of the surgery was approaching, but I still hadn't heard from the hospital about the time I should be there on operating day.

Back when I made the appointment, as it had been a last minute one, they told me I would get a phone call telling me what time to arrive. So the day before the surgery I decided to call the hospital myself. The receptionist was still waiting for the surgeon to give him the time, but he promised to get back to me before 5:00 p.m. Just a few minutes after that, the phone rang, and I was told to be at the hospital the next day at 2:00 p.m. for a 5:00 p.m. scheduled surgery. I was disappointed as I'd been hoping for a morning operation. Now I would have to fast until later, which meant by 5:00 p.m. I'd be a little weak.

On August 30, 2004, I arrived at the hospital early with Shoshi, Avi, and Yaniv. My daughter Orit was working at the deli to cover for us so she came a little later after she closed up. When filling out the forms, I listed Shoshi's name as my "in case of emergency person," and I sat down to wait for my name to be called. I looked around, noticing there were three more people waiting for surgery although it was 2:00 p.m. and I'd assumed that most surgeries were already finished. The room was very quiet, with all the occupants engrossed in their own thoughts.

When my name was called, Shoshi and I both got up, but the nurse stopped her, telling her she would be able to come in later. I was led to a long room filled with two rows of patients lying on beds. The nurse gave me a brown grocery bag and a hospital gown and pointed to the changing room. "Strip down and put on the gown," she said. "Use the bag for your clothes and personal belongings, and come out when you are ready. If you need to relieve yourself one last time before surgery, the toilet is behind the back door."

I came out of the restroom holding the brown bag and wearing the gown untied, because I couldn't reach the back to tighten it. I didn't care too much about it, but the nurse noticed my rear end was exposed, so she assisted me in tying the back of the gown. She asked me to lie down on the bed and wait for the anesthesiologist to come talk to me. While I was waiting, a different nurse came and took blood samples. To my right was a patient with an IV stand and all kind of wires hooked up to his body, and to my left was another patient in a similar situation.

My family soon came in; they took chairs and sat around me. Shoshi looked very worried. Some friends who'd arrived later also came in, but everyone was silent except for Yaniv, as it is in his nature to try to relax the atmosphere when it is too tense.

After an hour or so, the anesthesiologist came; he checked all the paperwork to verify that I was the intended patient, and then asked me what kind of anesthesia I preferred. I didn't expect that question as I thought it was a standard treatment. He told me I had a couple options: I could have conventional anesthesia, or I could have an epidural administered in my spine. As soon as Shoshi heard *epidural*, she jumped out of her chair and in a very determined voice said, "No epidural!" I assumed she associated it with giving birth and didn't want me to take any unnecessary risks. "Conventional," she said, answering for me.

The anesthesiologist walked away, and then the nurse came by. "I'll give you something to calm you down." To my surprise I was very calm, so I told her, "I don't need anything," but to no avail as she gave me the "something" anyway. The anesthesiologist returned with a student he was training, whom he asked to start the IV. After three failed attempts, the student successfully got the IV started.

I saw a few people in green robes walking up and down the room and asked, "Where is my surgeon?" "What do you need?" the anesthesiologist asked. "I just want to wish him good luck," I replied. They laughed and asked my family to leave, then rolled me down the hall to the operating room. The last thing I remember seeing before I lost consciousness was the table with the surgical tools being prepped by the medical team.

7
Recovery

I heard a lot of noise around me. I tried to open my eyes, and I managed to keep them open for a millisecond before I fell asleep again. When I woke up, I heard a lot of background noise, and from far away, I heard somebody saying, "He is trying to wake up." After what seemed like a long time, I heard noises again and opened my eyes for a little longer. I saw many people walking around. It felt like I was in the middle of a factory with equipment, noise, and lots of commotion.

Then I heard another voice saying, "He is trying to wake up again—why it is taking him so long?" It was very hard to keep my eyes open—no matter how hard I tried, I would suddenly sense nothing but quiet again. On the third attempt I managed to keep my eyes open. I wasn't sure where I was, but then I saw the green-robed people and my first thought was, "I'm alive!" What a great feeling that was. I felt a rush of adrenalin in my body, and I wanted to yell but I couldn't. I tried to move my head and my legs, but I couldn't do that either.

I heard a man saying, "He woke up." He asked, "How are you doing?" I nodded to indicate I was fine. "Your family is waiting outside—are you ready to see them?" I nodded again.

He started rolling the bed as I was examining myself. The first thing I noticed was I only had oxygen coming to my nose with no extra tubes. The instrument the nurse coordinator warned me about had come out before I woke up. I was elated by its absence, but although this small thing relieved me, I imagined I didn't look very good to anyone else. Then I thought about my family; we passed by a big clock, and I noticed it was 10:00 p.m. I had gone into surgery around 6:00 p.m., so my family had been waiting a long time to see me, and somehow I had to show them I was okay. The bed kept rolling and then the green-robed man said, "Here is your family." I turned to the right and they seemed so far away, it was as if they were on the other end of a football field. I managed to get my thumbs up from the sides of the bed, but I couldn't lift my hands and I wasn't sure if they would see it. But then I heard Yaniv saying, "He is giving us two thumbs up." It was a huge relief that they saw it, as now I could relax. The bed kept rolling, and I fell asleep again.

When I woke up, I was in the corner of a corridor with my family standing around me. I saw the green-robed man talking to the nurse in charge at the command post and handing her some paperwork. The responsibility for my recovery was now in the hands of the team in Department C, as I was in Room C 201-A.

I had a private corner room. Shoshi requested an extra bed so she could stay with me. At this point, I tried to persuade her that it was not necessary, but I was happy she did stay. The staff of doctors and nurses was wonderful, and they did all they could to help me recover fast, but it was Shoshi who gave me the minute-by-minute support and assistance that really helped me get better.

The progress was slow the first day. I felt a little better on the second day, but then a lot worse on the third. After the fourth day,

I was able to walk down the hallway, and from that point I started feeling stronger every day.

One day later that week, the nurse in charge came in and said, "You are taking a bath today." She helped me take my gown off and started cleaning my body with the special moist towels the hospital uses. She cleaned every part of me, changing towels in the process. "Here—take this towel and clean the area between your legs," she said. "Do you have shaving tools?" she asked in a commanding voice. "I don't feel like shaving," I replied. She responded, "You don't look good with a beard. I'll shave you"—and she did.

While she was doing so, she told me a story about a patient of hers she'd seen one day while Christmas shopping. When she stood behind him to pay, she'd said to him, "Hey, you look so much better with your clothes on!" not realizing that everybody was staring at her. I laughed—it's funny how what you are intending to say isn't always the same as what's being heard. After the bath and shave, I felt refreshed and clean. I looked much better, and more importantly, I felt much better.

I was discharged from the hospital one week after my operation, which included an exploratory laparotomy (a diagnostic procedure to assess disease in the abdomen) and a right hemicolectomy (removal of part of the colon). Before I left, I was instructed to make an appointment with Dr. W for a two-week postoperative follow-up. I stayed home one more week before resuming all my regular activities. I went back to work, and life started returning to normal again. My days once again began at the produce market at 5:00 a.m., where I would pick up the supply for the day, arriving at the deli around 6:00 a.m. and working until about 3:00 p.m.

On September 21, 2004, I went back to Stanford for my follow-up appointment with Dr. W. He told me that everything looked good, but I was still worried my blood tests weren't at the level they'd been before the surgery. Dr. W told me it would take time to get back to normal, so I should just continue to eat healthy and follow up with my physician after one year. He told me that my cancer (right colon) was only a Stage II, so I wouldn't need chemotherapy or radiation. I was very happy with the news, as I'd only heard of bad experiences with chemotherapy, and I was very encouraged when I learned I would be spared.

Before I left, I asked for all my medical records from my hospital stay so that I could add them to my binder. I was given a stack of papers, and I also asked Dr. W to send a report to my physician, Dr. S, so he would be informed when I went back to him for my follow-up visit. After thanking the medical team, I was on my way home.

As soon as I got there, I faxed all the medical records to my doctor friend in Indianapolis so he could give me additional feedback. Then I looked over all the reports myself. The clinic visit report read as follows: "Approximately one year from the date of his operation, we have instructed him to coordinate these follow-up studies with his primary care physician. Mr. Benaroya will not require a formal follow-up in our clinic. He is, however, encouraged to return if he desires or if any new problems arise."

8
The Big Dilemma

Dr. H works in an Indianapolis clinic next to a hospital. He received my fax in the clinic and took the papers home at the end of his day to look them over. Because of the different time zones (he's two hours ahead of me) and his long work day, it was close to midnight when he called me. I was very happy to hear his voice when I picked up the phone as I had many questions to ask, and he was the only professional I could consult without worrying I was offending or upsetting that person.

I wanted to know what he'd learned from the report, and he told me it looked like everything went well. However, I needed to focus on gaining my strength back to be ready for the next treatment. "Did they tell you when you are starting your chemotherapy?" he asked. "Oh no, they told me that I will not need any chemotherapy because my cancer was only Stage II," I replied. "The tumor went through the walls of the colon but didn't spread to any other organs."

Dr. H didn't agree with that conclusion at all, and he very strongly recommended I consult with a GI oncologist. When I tried to tell him I didn't want any chemo treatment because of all the side effects, he explained that colon cancer chemotherapy has only minor side effects, so I wouldn't even lose my hair. He recommended doing it as an insurance policy so that if any cancer was left in the colon, it would be killed by the chemo. Before we said good night to each other, my friend made me promise I would examine chemo as an option as he thought it was necessary.

The next day my brother from Israel called, and after the obvious questions about the state of my recovery, he also asked about my chemotherapy. As his wife runs a major medical center in Israel, he knows a thing or two about my illness. He told me that in Israel, regardless of the staging of the colon cancer, the standard treatment was surgery followed by chemo. He joined my doctor friend in Indianapolis in recommending I give it serious consideration.

I discussed the issue with Shoshi, and we agreed we needed to learn more about it. I went on the Internet and with the help of Google, read many articles on the subject, including those from the Web sites of Stanford Hospital, UCSF Hospital, and Mayo Clinic. What I learned from the research was that there are two schools of thought on whether chemotherapy should be recommended after Stage II colon cancer surgery. Now I had to decide which path I wanted to take.

It was a very difficult decision to make—I felt stronger every day, and a month afterwards, I'd almost forgotten I'd gone through such major surgery. Although I'd had some diarrhea the first few days after the operation, my bowel movements were now back to normal, and other than the scar on my abdomen, there were no signs I'd even had surgery. Starting chemo would cause my health to deteriorate, and I'd begin to lose my strength again.

After Shoshi and I talked it over, we decided against chemotherapy. My rationale was based on the fact that Dr. W, who had performed the surgery and was the only person to actually see my internal organs, told me I didn't need it. I should have complete confidence and trust in him in my healing process. The other factor influencing my decision was my philosophy regarding health. Shoshi and I believe medications should be used only on the rare occasion of a major illness. In our medicine cabinet you might find a few Band-Aids and maybe an expired bottle of Tylenol, but that was it. A headache wasn't reason enough to take medication as we felt it was better to tolerate the pain until it went away. We believe the more medication you take, the more you come to rely upon it, which means the body isn't as able to heal itself. Many people don't agree with this approach, but we felt very comfortable with it. So when we had to decide whether I should receive chemotherapy—which involves very toxic drugs—it was only natural for us to avoid it if possible, especially when my own doctor did not find it necessary.

At the time of my visit with Dr. W on September 21st, he'd asked me if I wanted to see an oncologist, and I declined. I must admit that as soon as I left the hospital, I had second thoughts about that, as another opinion couldn't have hurt. It is always a good idea to get as much information as possible before making this kind of serious decision. However, I was very set in my choice, and even Dr. H's attempts to persuade me to change my mind didn't influence it. He continued to call to check on my condition every week or two, and in every conversation he brought up the subject of chemo treatment. He never gave up trying to persuade Shoshi and me of its importance.

Because my decision was challenged so many times, I was no longer so sure I'd made the right one. Therefore, I didn't want to wait a year for a follow-up visit with my physician. Instead I decided to be more proactive and test more often so any problem would be detected earlier.

On October 10th, I called my physician's office and asked to take a blood test. The office manager promised she would talk to Dr. S and get back to me. She called back that afternoon and told me that I had a complete blood cell count (CBC) test order form ready to be picked up in the office. However, although Dr. S had agreed to order it, he thought it was still too soon after surgery.

The results came back after a couple of days, and they were very disappointing to me. Even though my hemoglobin and hematocrit results were within normal range (a low reading in these items usually indicates a blood loss), they were below my reading before I got sick (they were much higher at my 2000 physical exam). Yet because it had been only a little over a month since my surgery, it made sense to wait longer before having another test.

One month later I called the office again and this time requested a blood and stool test. On November 16, 2004, I received the report from the lab: my levels had slightly improved. I was satisfied to see an improvement in the blood area, but the stool test came back with two out of three samples positive for the presence of blood. This was very worrisome to me, but again as it was just over two months post-surgery, the blood in my stool could be caused by the surgery itself. After all, when organs are cut, there is bleeding, and there may have been some traces of blood still in my system—or at least that was my explanation.

When I shared this information with Dr. H, he recommended getting another test after six months and to also have a carcinoembryonic antigen (CEA) test that would indicate the presence of cancer cells. I agreed this was a good idea, but when December came around and we started planning a vacation, I wanted to have another test done then before traveling overseas.

Every year we closed our deli from Christmas through the year's end to take a vacation and give our employees some well-deserved time off. Our customers were accustomed to this tradition, and although they missed us, they were happy for us to have a chance to get away. It was always very exciting to come back in the new year and share our vacation experiences with them.

We generally went to Hawaii for our vacation because it's only a five-hour flight from California and it's a good place to go in December when temperatures are warm and the beaches are beautiful. (There aren't too many places close by us that have summer-like weather in the winter.) Another reason we liked going to Hawaii was our son Yaniv lived there, and he was happy to host us whenever we came.

However, this year we had a different trip planned: our daughter was studying abroad in London, so we decided to meet her in Greece for our vacation. Greece is my birth country, but I hadn't been back since my parents immigrated to Israel in 1953 when I was only five years old. I was really looking forward to this trip. My parents spoke Greek in our house when I was growing up, so I was able to retain most of the language. Going back to Greece more than fifty years later, I was excited about seeing what I'd remember from my childhood. The level of excitement was growing every day, but I couldn't ignore my health.

In mid-December I requested blood and stool tests again. To my disappointment, the results were not encouraging. There was deterioration in the blood readings, with both the hemoglobin and hematocrit being below normal range. On top of it all, three stool samples were positive. I was very frustrated by these results, but I wasn't going to ruin our trip to Greece. I'd wanted to go to back for a long time but had never planned anything. I felt that now was the time—I might not have another opportunity. I decided to put my health situation on hold until I returned.

9
A Break from It All

On December 22, 2004, Shoshi and I waited at a gate at San Francisco International Airport to board our KLM flight to Athens. Because I wasn't sure what my health would be like, I didn't plan our vacation much in advance. I'd placed a call to my relatives in Greece three weeks before our trip to get some guidance on where to stay in Athens. Immediately Lili and Yani Samaras offered to host us in their home. Our daughter Orit would meet us in Athens for her winter break from her studies in London. The offer was amazing, but I didn't know if they would have room for all of us, and I didn't want to impose. However, they insisted we spend the holidays with them, and we were very happy to accept.

Our flight had a ten-hour layover in Amsterdam, so when we arrived in the morning, we had some time to spare. We decided to take an organized tour of the city offered through one of the tourist booths outside of the airport. The flight from Amsterdam to Athens was very short, and after our luggage arrived, we walked toward the terminal exit where Lili was waiting to pick us up.

The meeting was slightly emotional: we hadn't seen Orit since she went to England five months earlier, and we hadn't seen the Samaras family since they moved back to Greece a few years back. From the airport Yani and Lili took us to their home in Kifysia, an upscale neighborhood in the suburbs of Athens. The house was beautiful and much larger than I'd anticipated. We were given our own room along with incredibly warm hospitality. The week to come was one of the best vacations of my life. I completely forgot about all my health problems and felt high on life.

Yani acted as our personal tour guide, and he was an excellent one. Of course we visited all the tourist attractions, but the highlights for me were traveling down memory lane. We visited the house in Plaka where I was born, and we saw the changing of the guards at the Parliament building, which hadn't changed from when my mother took me every day as a child. I stood there in awe for a long time, with flashbacks of many things I hadn't thought about since I was a child rushing through my mind. I was astonished at how many memories I had from the first five years of my life. I remembered a park where my mother used to take me whose name, *The Zapio*, was stuck in my mind. I mentioned the name to Yani, and in just a few phone calls he was able to find it. Once we got there, I realized the only thing I remembered about it was the name, but it was still great to see.

Lili and Yani were wonderful hosts; they took us anywhere I asked and gave us a complete tour of Athens. We saw the Acropolis, the taverns, the markets, and a whole lot more. They even took us to Pireus, where we boarded a ferry to one of the islands close by even though winter was not the island-hopping season.

The next leg of our trip began with a train ride to Thessalonica with my wife, daughter, and cousin Louisa. My father lived in Thessalonica for many years before he moved to Athens. He was the cofounder of the labor movement in Greece and very connected to Thessalonica. In 2002, my brother and I had been invited to Greece to attend a dedication ceremony of a hall in the labor union building that was being named after my father. Unfortunately I was unable to attend this event, but my younger brother went with his wife and had an amazing experience.

When we arrived in the city, it was decorated with lights for the holiday season, especially in the area of Aristotelous Square, which is downtown. The first thing I wanted to see was the labor union building and the hall dedicated to my father. I got the address from the front desk of our hotel, and we took a cab straight there. We arrived at the building a few minutes before 5:00 p.m., when there was only one person left in the building.

As we were about to enter, the man politely apologized and said they were about to close for the day. I identified myself as the son of Avraham Benaroya and asked if I could just go in for a few minutes to take a few photos. He very enthusiastically shook our hands and asked why we hadn't notified anyone of our arrival: "They could have at least cleaned the place up and had someone there to greet you!" He smiled and welcomed us in, then gave us a tour of the building. As we entered the Benaroya Hall I saw a huge banner with my father's picture hanging from the ceiling; his photograph was surrounded by different quotes from his speeches. We took many photos of the building and signs and thanked the man for his kindness. On our way out he gave us a stack of books and articles he had about my father.

Our next stop in Thessalonica was the Jewish Museum. After going through the security screening, we went upstairs to view the exhibits. Thessalonica was the home of a large Jewish community that perished during the Holocaust. The museum exhibits reflected the central role the Jews played in the community at large. On the wall were photos of local leaders, among them one of my father.

From the museum we went to the famous local market that probably looked exactly the same as it did when my father used to shop there for produce and fish. After a few more extraordinary days in Thessalonica, we took a long train ride back to Athens. The trip to Thessalonica was the highlight of my visit as it was remarkable to see my father's presence in this town more than half a century after he'd left.

When the train arrived in Athens, Yani was waiting for us at the station. We hurried home to shower and rest before attending a Greek New Year's party with Lili and Yani's friends. The party was the perfect end to our trip, with excellent Greek food and wonderful people. The next morning we boarded our plane back to San Francisco and the reality waiting for us there.

10
Back to Reality

For most people, the expression "back to reality" after a nice vacation means going back to work or school; for me that reality was very different. Not only did I have to go back to work, but I had to revisit my medical situation. There were many questions wandering through my mind: Was I free of my cancer? Did I have something else wrong with me this time? Had my iron deficiency problem been resolved? I needed to find the answers.

I placed a call to my physician's office to request another blood test. On January 5, 2005, I got the report: both hemoglobin and hematocrit were below normal levels. It had now been four months since my surgery and all the signs were still worrisome. The stool test results were even worse than the blood tests—all three samples came back positive. In general I was feeling good, but my report card did not reflect that.

I called for a family meeting to try to figure out my next step. Yaniv recommended we call my surgeon, Dr. W, for advice. The next day Yaniv left a message for Dr. W, who called back within an hour. After hearing the outcome of my tests, he expressed his confidence that the surgery had been successful. However, he suggested I call the GI doctor who had performed my colonoscopy to get his opinion, implying that something might have been missed during the colonoscopy.

The GI doctor was not cooperative at all—as a matter of fact, he was very rude. The way he put it, he'd done a good job, and he was sure that everything was okay. He then raised his voice to express his opinion about the habits of Jewish people: "They always like to worry!" he shouted. Before hanging up the phone, he kept yelling, "What do you want from me?" He wouldn't even listen to what I was saying; instead he was immediately angry and defensive and didn't even try to calm or reassure me. We were in complete shock, as the fact he was also Jewish didn't give him any right to behave in such an unprofessional manner.

Now we were facing a new dilemma: I couldn't go back to this GI doctor, but I didn't know anybody else to trust. I decided to call my surgeon again. I spoke with the nurse coordinator, and although she was very kind and sympathetic, she couldn't help much. She told me I needed to see a GI doctor as there wasn't much that my surgeon could do at that point. I explained to her I had lost trust in my GI doctor and asked if she could recommend someone else to me. She promised to call back before 5:00 p.m., and she kept her promise. She referred me to Dr. L, an associate professor at Stanford. I didn't want to waste any time, so I called right away to make an appointment. To my surprise, after I described my problem, I was able to get an appointment for the very next day.

Dr. L was very pleasant and friendly, and I immediately liked him. He made an effort to get to know me, asking about my occupation and family. I told him about the deli I owned with my wife, and he told me about his father's restaurant. He knew a lot about the food business, and the small talk helped relax me a bit. When he asked for my medical records, I handed him my entire binder. He spent a few minutes looking through my records, especially focusing on the GI report and the photos of my colonoscopy.

"Does it look like cancer?" I asked in a doubtful voice about the tumor that was previously removed. "Oh yes," he replied. "This is cancer." He asked about my last GI doctor, but I didn't offer much information and he dropped the subject quickly. He then put gloves on and proceeded with the examination, including a rectal exam in which he tested for the presence of blood. "This is the dirty part of my job," he said. "You are bleeding from somewhere, and most times the source of bleeding is either the colon or the stomach. Since the tumor in your colon was removed, it could be ulcers causing the bleeding."

There were two ways to find the source of my bleeding. The first option was for me to swallow a capsule containing a built-in camera that would record everything in its path until it exited my body. When Dr. L told me about this option, I remembered reading about it. The second was for me to have my stomach looked at endoscopically. This procedure uses a probe with a little camera on it that enters the body through the mouth. Through it, Dr. L could look for any abnormalities in my stomach. If nothing was found as a result of these procedures, the next step would be another colonoscopy to look at things from the opposite end.

Per his recommendation, I agreed to the endoscopy followed by the colonoscopy. According to Dr. L, the camera pill option was not very accurate because it flips in the system resulting in many blank spots.

However, when I tried to schedule the appointment with Dr. L's assistant, she told me his schedule was completely booked. Luckily, Dr. L insisted she squeeze me in somewhere, so she found me an opening for January 12, 2005, at 10:00 a.m.

Suddenly I found myself sitting in front of a registration window once again, waiting with Shoshi for my second colonoscopy within six months. To prepare for it, I had to drink a bottle of Fleet the night before to clean out my colon. The Fleet was even more disgusting than I remembered, and after the first dose, I couldn't imagine taking the second. It took me twenty minutes just to finish drinking the first six-ounce cup, and it didn't take long to kick in. I went to the bathroom so many times that I was sure there was nothing left in me, and I wrongly assumed I could get away with only one dose. I later realized I'd made a big mistake.

As I was waiting nervously in my chair, the nurse called my name and I jumped out of my seat. Before following her into the exam room, I whispered to Shoshi, "I hope it goes fast." It was anything but that. After I filled out all the paperwork and answered many questions, they started the IV on my arm and left me in a bed waiting for a room. The procedure before mine was taking much longer than scheduled, so I had to wait a while. Finally I saw the door to the exam room open and a patient rolled out on a bed. It was my turn next.

Before I was taken into the room, I saw Dr. L pick a tool that looked like a garden hose from a wall of many different-sized hoses. I hoped he picked the right size, as I had no idea how a doctor determined the size of someone's colon. After I saw him grab my hose and I was brought into the room, I began to mentally prepare myself for the colonoscopy.

Because I had only been thinking of the colonoscopy, I had completely forgotten the first procedure would involve inserting an instrument via my mouth. Dr. L sprayed my tongue with some medication to sedate the area, and then inserted the apparatus through my mouth and down my throat. To my surprise, it didn't choke me at all. The exam only took a few minutes and ended with a little discomfort, but no findings.

Then I turned on my side for the second invasion. The colonoscopy took much longer than my first one, but I didn't find out why until after the exam. After almost an hour, I was taken out of the exam room and placed in a side room to wait for the report.

Dr. L returned after some time with a written report and photos that had been taken from the inside of my colon. "Do you see this dark thing here?" he asked. "This is stool that should have left your system if you had drunk the Fleet last night. Did you drink it?" I shamefully admitted taking only one dose. "You made my job more difficult, but I managed to take two samples from the anastomosis area." That was the area where my colon was reconnected after my surgery. He told me it felt a little bumpy, and he would let me know the results of the biopsy as soon as he received them.

He then gave me his pager number and told me to call if I had any questions. I was stunned—I'd never been given a pager number by any doctor. After my experience with the first GI doctor, I now felt like I was in very good hands.

I felt much better after my second colonoscopy than I did after the first. I was happy there was no obvious cancerous tumor, and there was a chance the biopsy could come back benign.

Four days after the colonoscopy, Dr. L called with the biopsy results. He spoke quickly but very empathetically: "I just received the biopsy report, and both samples came back positive. I'm very sorry—it came as a surprise to me. I did not expect it to be malignant."

I could not believe my ears. It was barely six months since my surgery, and I had just been informed I had colon cancer once again. I didn't understand it because I was told that colon cancer was very slow growing, but now after recovering from my surgery, I was back at square one. "How could this happen?" I asked him. He sounded puzzled himself. "I really don't know," he said. "I'm sorry that you have to go through this again."

"Is this a new tumor? Was it missed during the surgery? Where did it come from?" I was full of questions, but Dr. L didn't have the answers. "So what do I do?" I asked.

"You need to have another surgery. I've already sent all the information to Dr. W," he replied. I was in a complete state of shock and didn't know what to think. I couldn't help but feel I was missing part of the story.

It was a little late at night, but I decided to call Dr. H to get some answers. He was as shocked as I was. "I've been a GI doctor for thirty years, and I have never heard of a case where a tumor in the colon came back in six months. I think it is more likely that you had another tumor that was missed the first time around, but I still don't understand it. I know Stanford is an excellent hospital, and it's hard for me to believe that they would miss a tumor."

I hesitated slightly before I asked. "Did the fact I didn't have chemotherapy have anything to do with it?" "Not likely," he replied. "Six months isn't long enough for a recurrence—it takes much longer for a tumor to develop. But this time you must do chemotherapy after surgery!" He raised his voice. "You must!" he repeated. He reassured me that the treatment was not too strong and that I would only need adjuvant chemotherapy, which would involve no hair loss. At this point I couldn't even accept that I needed a second surgery, so chemotherapy was the furthest thing from my mind. I agreed to thoroughly visit all my options before making any decisions and said good night to Dr. H.

The next day I called my physician, Dr. S, to inform him of my situation. He was just as surprised as everyone else. I asked for his opinion on the likelihood that it was a new growth versus something left behind during the surgery. Without hesitation he said it had most likely been overlooked the first time around. I then asked if he could recommend a surgeon, and he once again referred me to the "local talent," as he put it, which was Dr. R, the surgeon I'd seen first but whose appointment I'd canceled to switch to Dr. W. I detected in his tone of voice that Dr. S was somewhat disappointed with my decision to choose Stanford for my treatment over the local hospital. I thanked him for his time, and I requested another blood and stool test, as I still hadn't accepted the outcome from the first one.

On January 28, 2005, the test results indicated an improvement in my blood count, but all three stool samples came back positive for the presence of blood. I was slightly encouraged by the improvement in the blood cell count. Even though my levels were still below my pre-surgery levels, they were now within normal range. I began to look for reasons for the blood in my stool as I still wasn't ready to accept that I had cancer *again*. I thought that maybe the blood was there because I'd gone to the dentist a few days before I took the samples, and that maybe when I bled in my mouth, it affected my stool. I called my dentist for answers, but to my disappointment he dismissed the idea immediately.

On January 30th, I had a CT scan at Stanford that Dr. L ordered after the biopsy results came back. I was secretly hoping the CT scan would prove that everything was okay and the biopsy was in error. But obviously that was not the reason for the test. I waited to see Dr. W with Shoshi and Yaniv by my side. We were in a very crowded room, and every time the nurse opened the door to call a name, my stress level escalated. A woman was giving free massages in the waiting room, and people kept adding their names to the list. I thought about doing so, but the list was way too long. So instead of the massage, I started pacing up and down the hallway.

Finally the door opened and the nurse called my name. The three of us followed her inside. The now familiar process began—my blood pressure, weight, and temperature were taken, and we were led to Dr. W's treatment room. The nurse put my file in the slot on the door and requested we wait for the doctor.

After what seemed like a very long time, a group of medical students came in. I recognized the one in charge as he had been there during my last visit just a few months earlier. He looked through my file but avoided making eye contact with us. He expressed both his and Dr. W's surprise to see us back so soon. He, like everyone else, told us they didn't understand what had happened. After asking me a few questions, he left the room and told us that Dr. W would be in shortly. The entire time he was in the room, he didn't make eye contact with any of us. I was very distraught, and Shoshi and the children felt the same way.

Dr. W came in after a while, and he also expressed his surprise at seeing me back in the clinic so soon. Judging from his body language and tone of voice, it was an uncomfortable situation for him, but for me it was very disturbing. He offered an explanation for the newly discovered tumor. Unlike the other theories of it being left behind, he said it was possible that there were some floating cancerous cells left in my colon after the surgery, and they could have reestablished themselves at the anastomosis. When he performed the surgery, he took a five-centimeter margin from each side of the tumor, and the biopsy report came back clean, so this was the only explanation he could think of. When he saw the skeptical looks on our faces, especially mine, he suggested we get a second opinion, so he referred us to the surgeon at UCSF who'd taken over Dr. W's position when he moved to Stanford.

I didn't like Dr. W's explanation of my tumor, feeling he was blaming my body rather than the surgery or colonoscopy. It would have been easier for me to accept the prospect of a second surgery if I knew the second tumor was missed earlier and not something that had just developed in six months. If my body was producing tumors that fast, I thought there would be no point in my having surgery only to have to return six months later for a repeat. I knew that colons were very long, but if I had to cut a piece out every six months, I would run out of colon fairly quickly. I left Dr. W's office a little frustrated, but I agreed to make an appointment to see the San Francisco surgeon.

We went downstairs to pick up the CT film and make the arrangements to send the specimens from the colonoscopy to the UCSF laboratory for a second evaluation. When we arrived home, I decided to call my friend Dr. H for advice. He supported getting a second opinion, but he warned me not to expect anything different. As for why Dr. W wasn't considering the possibility of something being missed during surgery, Dr. H explained the medical establishment has become a target for endless lawsuits, and doctors have to be very careful of what they admit to in order to protect themselves.

I'm not the suing type, and it's hard for me to imagine people suing the persons who are trying to save their lives. After all, we are all human, and even if a mistake had been made, it would be much easier for me to accept than the alternative. I'm sure there are some cases in which legal action is necessary, but it should only happen if there is intentional negligence, and with criminal intent. For example, if my surgeon came in to work intoxicated and amputated a healthy leg, then I might be inclined to sue. I think it's very sad that America has become such a litigation-happy society as ultimately, we are all paying for it. Throughout my treatments, I never had a doubt that my medical team members were doing everything they could to save my life.

A few days later I went to see the UCSF surgeon; he was very nice, but, as expected, he couldn't tell me anything different. After giving me a thorough examination, looking at the images from the CT scan, and reading the biopsy report that was reevaluated at the UCSF laboratory, he concluded a floating cell or cells regrouped after my surgery and formed a new tumor. His only recommendation was surgery. He also mentioned to me that his methods were very similar to Dr. W's, with the only difference being how they reconnected the colon after a section was removed. He connected the two ends of the colon using stitches, whereas Dr. W used a system of pins. He praised Dr. W, but said he would be happy to do my surgery if that were my wish.

Before leaving I asked him if he knew of any way to solve my problem without surgery, and he recommended consulting with the homeopathic department at UCSF. At first it seemed like a good idea to check it out, but due to the rapid growth of my tumor, Shoshi and I thought it would be too risky to experiment at this stage with less proven methods of treatment.

I tried to keep an open mind to all ideas, and I appreciated everything being presented to me. On the way home Shoshi and I discussed the situation and agreed to seek a third opinion. We decided that if there was consensus among three different doctors, we would follow that path. We called the children to inform them of our decision and to collaborate to find another surgeon. Avi found a site that evaluated doctors on several different parameters, and sent me the link to www.healthgrades.com. After looking at this site, he recommended we schedule an appointment with a colorectal surgeon from Concord, California, who had twenty years of experience in the field.

Coincidentally, the father of one of Avi's employees happened to be a colorectal surgeon at Stanford. Avi offered to call him for a consultation, and it seemed like a good idea. He spoke with Avi for over an hour, and he came to the same conclusion: I needed surgery, and he was available to do it if I wanted. Apparently Avi did such a good job describing my condition that he didn't need to see me or any medical records to recommend surgery.

Yaniv flew in from Hawaii once again, and on February 16th he came with me to see the Concord surgeon, Dr. O. When the doctor entered the examination room, I was lying on the bed with my gown on. He looked at my scar from the surgery and asked who had diagnosed me. I told him Dr. L had done so after performing a colonoscopy and ordering a biopsy. "Why did you go to a GI so soon after your surgery?" he wondered. "Well, I requested blood and stool tests from my physician, and when the results weren't ideal, I went to Dr. L." "So you are the one who diagnosed your problem," he replied, crediting me with the diagnosis.

He continued, "You have another problem though—has anyone told you that you have a hernia? Put your hand on your crotch and cough." I felt my bones moving. "Remember, I'm the one who diagnosed your hernia. Now dress up and meet me in the office."

When I was ready, Yaniv and I closed the door behind us and sat down, anxious to hear what the doctor had to say. "You have a problematic colon. I recommend removing the colon completely and connecting the small intestine to the rectum. By doing this, you could avoid the chance of recurrence. If you agree, I can schedule you for next week. The only problem is that you would have permanent diarrhea for the rest of your life." I was not a fan of his hard closing tactics, and I wasn't ready to lose my colon yet.

After this last consult, I realized the best thing for me would be to have the surgery with Dr. W. Aside from the tumor coming back, I was very happy with him the first time around, and I figured he had the most invested in my case. I was comfortable with the staff at Stanford, and even if he did make a mistake the first time, I was sure he wouldn't repeat it. Although I was obviously still not happy with my diagnosis, I realized I needed the surgery, and I wanted Dr. W to perform it. The only thing left to do was to call Dr. W's office and schedule a date.

The next day I called his nurse coordinator, requesting mine be the first surgery of the day. The first time, not only did I have a long fast because mine was the last surgery of the day, but I also worried my surgeon had been tired after a long day of work. To my satisfaction, my request was granted, and I was told to be at the hospital at 6:00 a.m. on February 28, 2005.

11
The Second Surgery

Another issue we had to deal with was our business. We had owned the deli for sixteen years and enjoyed the work we were doing, but it had become apparent my return to normal work hadn't contributed to my recovery, and maybe the opposite was true. Therefore, we made the decision to put our deli up for sale. It was very hard for Shoshi to accept our closing this chapter of our lives, but she understood its necessity. Fortunately, we had been able to put aside retirement money that was invested well to give us a reasonable standard of living. And Shoshi, if she wanted, could always find work in the field she loved. Meanwhile, we would need help again while Shoshi spent time with me at the hospital. Yaniv stepped up to the plate and agreed to cover for both of us. Fortunately, the deli was now the responsibility of the new owner, but we had to provide training for one month, and Yaniv and Orit took care of this obligation.

At 6:00 a.m. on February 28, 2005, I checked in for surgery at Stanford Hospital. The night before I'd completed the system clean-up procedure, this time making sure to consume the full dose of the medication as I didn't need any complications during surgery. I was already familiar with the bureaucracy, and everything went quickly and smoothly.

However, while I was sitting down waiting for my name to be called, I tried to read the newspaper, but I couldn't focus. I flipped the pages, reading only the headlines before putting it down. I ended up sitting silently, without exchanging words with Shoshi until I heard my name being called. I knew exactly where to go. Shoshi stayed behind as they would bring her in later with the rest of the family and friends after I was prepared for surgery.

As I was changing out of my clothes and into the hospital gown, I was thinking about the conversation I'd had with Dr. W during the clinic visit before the day of surgery. Dr. W had told us he'd discussed my condition with Dr. L, and they both agreed the possibility of a tumor being left in the colon during the first surgery was real. This made me feel better about my decision to repeat the surgery. I didn't see any point of going through this every six months if my body insisted on growing tumors.

The surgery went well but took longer this time. Later I read in the surgeon's report there was a large amount of omentum (fatty tissue) attached to the colon that had taken some time to clear. I was moved to the same unit where everybody was surprised to see me again. My recovery was very quick: Shoshi again stayed in my room for the duration of my hospitalization, providing love and care during my time of need. The wonderful hospital staff made it possible for my stay to be only one week; I could continue my recovery at home.

In the beginning I was walking daily in our backyard for ten minutes at a time, and as I gained strength, I increased the walking time by going around the block. By the fourth week I was walking for half an hour a day and starting to gain back some of the weight I'd lost.

Shoshi was going to work every day at 5:00 a.m., covering my shift, and getting home around 6:00 p.m. This was very hard for her, but fortunately she wouldn't have to do it for long. After the new owner's one month of training was completed, we would have a lot of time to spend together.

We were looking forward to some time alone. I felt strong again, and we agreed taking a trip abroad was the right thing to do now. I had a follow-up appointment with Dr. W in mid-April, so we decided to make our travel plans after we got a good health report.

12
More Time Off

On April 20, 2005, we departed from San Francisco for a two-month vacation starting in Oahu, Hawaii, and continuing on to Japan, Thailand, Cambodia, Maui, and the Big Island of Hawaii. This was our first time ever taking this long of a vacation and visiting new places. Previously, our longest vacation was two weeks with the overseas destinations being Israel or Greece, where we have family. We were looking forward to learning about different cultures and visiting all the tourist sites.

After a two-week stay in Honolulu with Yaniv spent relaxing on the beach, the three of us flew to Tokyo. The airport was an hour's train ride away from downtown. After we arrived at our destination and got off, we found ourselves in a huge station crammed with people with exits all over the place. We picked one of them randomly and looked for somebody to ask about hotel directions. We saw a lady walking toward us, obviously in a hurry. We stopped her, hoping she spoke some English. She didn't, but using hand signals, she expressed her willingness to help.

Tokyo is a city with many skyscrapers and neon lights that slightly resembles Las Vegas, but I was mostly impressed with the helpful attitude of its people. Our first experience was repeated throughout our stay. We used the train system to move around, with there being six to ten trains at a time stopping at the station. All we needed to do was show someone our destination and the person would escort us to the train we needed to take. Not one time did we get lost using the train system in Tokyo. We were told the trains are never late and that we could actually adjust our watches according to the train arrival and departure time.

The Tokyo streets were always crowded with people, and the crosswalks were very wide to accommodate the large numbers. The level of pollution was high, and we saw many people wearing face masks for protection. At one time I considered purchasing a mask for myself, but I didn't want to waste too much time—after all, we were only spending a week there, so I expected my lungs to survive the poor air quality.

Satisfied we'd managed to see all that we had planned in Japan in one short week, we next traveled to Bangkok, Thailand. We found out that when you book a hotel online, it's not so easy to tell if the location is what you want. Ours was in a poor neighborhood with many street merchants selling everything from food items displayed without any refrigeration or with only minimal sanitation to designer-label suits. Everything was quite cheap, but I was very concerned about the food as with my condition, I couldn't afford any problems. We tried to eat in what looked like relatively clean places, hoping for the best. Shoshi couldn't resist the low prices, so we spent too much time shopping.

The one thing I took advantage of was the famous Thai massage, especially the foot massage. An hour-long reflexology massage was only five dollars and included a map of your foot showing what organs in the body are controlled by what area on it. My son, who had persuaded me in the first place to try the Thai massage (it was my first massage *ever*), pointed out to me that according to the diagram, this massage can do a lot to improve a person's sex life. However, at that time my organ of focus was my colon for obvious reasons, and I asked the masseuse to concentrate on that area. I could use any help I could get for a healthy colon, and to this day Thai massage has been the only enjoyable medical treatment I've received.

Orit joined us from Chiang Mai, where she was attending school, for the next leg of our trip: Cambodia. We flew there in a small plane, which did not make me feel safe at all. I was relieved when after an hour or so, we landed safely. When we exited the terminal, a fleet of private cars waited to serve the transportation needs of tourists. As there are no taxis in this area, many car owners use their vehicles to earn a living. We were assigned a young driver who spoke sufficient English to make communication manageable. After our experience with hotels in Thailand, I didn't have high expectations for the "four-star" hotel we'd reserved prior to our arrival, but to my surprise the hotel was new and very modern. This is because of Angkor Wat, the amazingly preserved ruins of the twelfth-century temples that attract many people. To accommodate the growing number of tourists, the government has built new hotels on a strip of land surrounded by low-income housing.

Our driver offered to serve us for the duration of our stay as well as provide a government-licensed guide fluent in English. We didn't regret accepting the offer as the guide was well informed and had a pleasant personality. The two of them never left us during our three-day visit to Cambodia. The driver slept in the car at night in the hotel parking lot to ensure no one would take our business from him. We spent one day touring the Angkor Wat ruins with the help of our guide. I was fascinated with the history, temples, and architecture, and this was definitely the highlight of the Asian trip for me.

We flew back to Bangkok, where we spent two additional days before returning to Honolulu. After a two-day rest at Yaniv's home, Shoshi and I continued to the next destination: the island of Maui, where we had friends who hosted us very warmly for three days. We enjoyed their company and familiarity with the island, and we visited the most beautiful sites that only the locals know.

The last stop of our long vacation was the Big Island of Hawaii, where we rented a car and drove from Kona to Hilo with the highlight being the volcano watch of Kilauea. The flow of lava to the Pacific Ocean is visible at night with hundreds of visitors gathering to observe this spectacular sight from a safe distance. It was a beautiful ending to a long and enjoyable trip. On Sunday, June 5, 2005, we returned to San Francisco International Airport.

13
Monitoring Continues

During the whole trip I felt very good, and I didn't have any reason to suspect any health problems. After a short rest I resumed my physical activity, mainly walking for one hour a day and slowly increasing the time. On the weekends Motty and I started going to Lake Chabot again for a four- to five-mile walk. However, because of my health history, I remained very vigilant about any signs of trouble. During every visit to the restroom, I inspected the toilet paper for traces of blood, did excessive stretching exercises to make sure I didn't get dizzy, and in general watched for any abnormalities. This didn't mean I became paranoid or a hypochondriac, only that I was on guard.

Often I spoke with my doctor friend in Indianapolis, who reassured me I should be fine and that two surgeries shouldn't negatively affect my life expectancy. He repeated that colon cancer is one of the slowest-growing cancers and that, if detected early, a full recovery is expected. However, every time we talked, Dr. H would remind me I needed to see an oncologist and start chemotherapy as an insurance policy. I was very uncomfortable telling him I'd decided not to do it, so instead every time the subject came up, I would promise to look for a good oncologist in my area. I did call my brother in Israel, who with the help of his wife found a renowned oncologist in San Francisco, but I never called him. Dr. H never gave up trying to persuade me of the necessity of getting chemotherapy started. I later regretted not listening to him.

Shoshi started talking about the possibility of getting a part-time job to keep herself busy and earn some money. She is a very energetic person, and retirement at this juncture didn't appeal to her very much. Avi owns an online swim outlet that employs about fifty people, and when he extended an offer to her to work twice a week as a company chef, she promised to consider it.

We entered the month of July, and Shoshi decided to celebrate my recovery by sending out invitations for a big birthday party for me on the 31st. I wanted to have an added cause for celebration, so I requested a blood test to see if I had reached the pre-cancer blood count levels. The report from the lab came two days before the party: my hemoglobin and hematocrit levels were within the normal ranges, but a little below the levels of the previous test taken on April 12th. I didn't worry about it very much because all the variables, such as how much water I drank and what I ate, can make a difference in blood counts—something I'd learned from the lab nurse.

On Sunday, July 31st, we celebrated my birthday with all our friends. I felt very lucky to have such a wonderful wife who took care of me when I was sick and had organized a great party with excellent food and good friends, something that only she knows how to do. I felt very happy—we had probably fifty to sixty guests, and they had a good time. On the following Monday morning at breakfast, I thanked Shoshi for the party, and she said how much she'd enjoyed doing it and that she was thinking of accepting Avi's offer to work two days a week. I encouraged her to do so, as I knew she missed the deli, and working for our son sounded like a winning idea.

A week went by, and I started thinking again about the last blood test I'd taken. Now it no longer made sense to me that the reading hadn't improved, and that in fact the opposite was true. I decided to ask for a stool test because I wanted to make sure I was okay before Shoshi went back to work. I called my physician's office and requested one. They called me back after few hours to let me know that Dr. S had approved the test even though he didn't think it was necessary.

The next day I picked up the test package that contained the three special envelopes for three samples I needed to collect on different days. I did so and delivered the kit to the lab on August 16th. Three days later the dreaded phone call came: all three samples tested positive for the presence of blood. I asked, "Are you sure?" in disbelief, and the answer was yes. For a few minutes, I didn't know what to say, and then I asked for the report to be faxed to me. The report read positive three times in the out-of-range column. There was no possibility of a mistake; all the samples were taken on different days, and all of them were positive. It wasn't good news.

I shared the results with Shoshi, who took this development very badly, immediately calling the children. Wondering what my next step should be, I decided to fax the report to my GI specialist, Dr. L. Five minutes later the phone rang, and Dr. L was on the other end of the line. "Somebody faxed me this report," he began, obviously not recognizing my name. "Yes, it was me," I replied, identifying myself. He immediately remembered and asked me about the trip to Israel we'd planned before my second surgery but had to cancel. I was surprised he remembered as after all, some time had passed since I'd told him about it. "We are planning to leave on September 15th," I said. "But now these stool test results—what should I do?"

After a long silence, he said he would do a colonoscopy. "It is a coincidence that you found me in the clinic. I'm on a sabbatical right now, but I will do your colonoscopy. My assistant will call you to schedule an appointment." "Should I cancel my trip?" I asked. "Definitely not. I'm doing it just to prove to you that everything is okay. There must be some other explanation." I thanked him for his quick response and his willingness to see me during his sabbatical, but I was not convinced I was okay.

On Wednesday, August 31st, one month after my birthday, we arrived at Stanford Hospital for my third colonoscopy in a single year. I couldn't help thinking about my first one in August 2004 and my doubts about its necessity. Since then I'd learned that if I'd had a colonoscopy when I turned fifty, there was a good chance I wouldn't be in this predicament. As I learned from Dr. F's speech at a colon cancer survivors conference held at Stanford Hospital, one of the sad statistics about colonoscopy is that only a small percentage of the population in the United States uses this screening method, which can *prevent* colorectal cancer. This is in comparison with the much larger percentage of women who receive mammograms for early detection of breast cancer. The difference here is early detection compared with prevention. I was one of these statistics as I thought it couldn't happen to me.

Dr. L is an experienced GI doctor, and he didn't need to wait for the pathology report to advise me that our trip to Israel would have to be postponed until a later time. He explained to us that my situation was very unusual; in fact, he hadn't heard of any similar case of recurrent colorectal cancer on the anastomosis. In response to my question as to the need for another operation, he said that because of the unique case I represented, he would have to consult with a number of doctors to determine the best course of action. He would present my case to what he called the tumor board, which consists of a group of surgeons, oncologists, GI physicians, and other specialists who would discuss the situation and recommend a treatment.

I wasn't surprised about the findings: in a phone conversation I'd had the day before with Yaniv, when he asked me what I thought was the cause of the bleeding, I'd told him that probably my body for some unknown reason was insisting on growing tumors. My thoughts were clear, and I didn't panic, but I knew one of the possibilities was that I could die. To my big surprise, I wasn't afraid. I accepted the fact because as I saw it, my body had made a mistake and grown a cancer cell. It was my body's job to correct that mistake, and I was going to do all I could to help. Dr. L expressed his sorrow for my situation and scheduled the tumor board appointment for the beginning of the following week.

We arrived home in the late afternoon. Shoshi was very distressed, and I did not feel that great ether. We called the children to give them the news. Yaniv decided to book a flight home, as he wanted to be present at my appointment with the tumor board. Next, I called Dr. H in Indianapolis to inform him of the situation and get his opinion. He was totally shocked; he also had never heard of a case like this, and he tried to lift my spirits. To my question of whether the lack of chemotherapy was to blame, he answered probably not, but I knew then I'd made a mistake. I decided not to think about what I could have done but concentrate on the best action from that point forward.

According to Dr. H, another surgery was inevitable, but I should wait to hear the conclusion of the tumor board before even thinking about it. He also promised to inquire about my case with all his colleagues around the world and call me back with the findings.

That night I had a hard time falling asleep. My brain was searching for answers. How could I help my body correct this terrible mistake it had made without having to go through another surgery? I remember vividly thinking that if I could help it, I had to make sure this would not be a fatal mistake.

14
The Three Options

The next day while I was preparing my medical records binder for the tumor board appointment, the television was on and I overheard the word *cancer*. From that point on, I stopped everything I was doing to watch a full interview of a medical doctor who had breast cancer and said she'd been cured without surgery by using only alternative medicine. I was very interested in what she had to say. According to her, she'd been near death using conventional medicine, and only after she changed to alternative medicine was she cured. I listened very carefully when she claimed the only reason people get sick is because of a weak immune system, and the main reason for that is dehydration. Simply put, we don't drink enough water. Only at the end of this interview when a toll-free telephone number appeared on the screen did I realize that what I was watching was an infomercial. Dr. Lorraine Day was promoting her tapes, and the one I was watching was called "Cancer Doesn't Scare Me Anymore."

I didn't waste any time in calling to order the tape. In a nutshell, the message was that cancer is not caused by a lack of chemotherapy or radiation, and therefore they can't be used as treatments for cancer. Chemotherapy and radiation actually cause cancer. Surgery, which she called mutilation, was also not the answer. No surgery, no chemotherapy—that was exactly what I wanted to hear. Her credentials were impressive: she had been an orthopedic trauma surgeon for fifteen years and both an associate professor and vice chair of the Department of Orthopedic Surgery at the UCSF School of Medicine. She was also chief of orthopedic surgery at San Francisco General Hospital.

As I watched the tapes over and over, I couldn't help thinking about the huge responsibility she was taking on by selling those tapes. When I tried to call for an appointment with her, I was told she doesn't give any personal consultations. Apparently she makes enough money selling the tapes. I couldn't disagree with most of her remedies: drinking enough water, breathing fresh air outdoors, and having an attitude of gratitude all sounded like good things. But to completely abandon conventional medicine was a little too extreme for me.

On September 14, 2005, Shoshi, Yaniv, and I arrived at the Stanford Hospitals and Clinics for the appointment with the tumor board. We were led to a room at the end of a corridor where a number of doctors were gathered. The nurse asked a few questions and then explained the procedure of the tumor board. I thought I was the only one to be discussed at the meeting, but apparently there were a number of cases on the agenda with mine being only one of them.

When I showed the nurse my medical binder containing a year's worth of medical records, she seemed surprised I had such a thing. She asked to borrow it for board use, and I gladly gave it to her, hoping it would be used. She then told us that the time scheduled for the board was between two and three hours and we were free to go and come back in two hours to that room. We decided to use the time to have lunch at the hospital cafeteria.

When we came back after two hours, the board was not finished deliberating. It was another hour before we saw the door open and a large number of doctors walk out. Dr. W came directly to our room. I was nervous and felt like I was in a courtroom drama at the point when the jury is about to read the verdict. I could see in Dr. W's eyes that I had better be prepared for some tough realities.

He began by telling me how interesting my case was—unfortunately for me. They didn't understand why I had a different biology than most people, and not only did they not have a similar case in their hospital, but he didn't know of a case like mine anywhere. That's great, I thought to myself, I always wanted to be special, but not in that way.

Dr. W proceeded with giving me the three options the tumor board recommended for my treatment. Option number one, which ensured the least risk of recurrence, was a total colectomy and proctectomy with an ileostomy. In layperson's terms, it meant the total removal of the colon, anus, and rectum, bringing the small intestine out through the abdomen in order to collect the waste material in an outside bag. Option number two was to connect the small intestine to the rectum (iliorectal anastomosis). This option provided the advantage of a normal outside appearance, but at the risk of a higher chance of recurrence and a lifelong battle with diarrhea and occasional leaks. Option number three was resecting the tumor with an ileal pouch–anal anastomosis, which involved removing the colon and rectum while preserving the anus and sphincter muscles and creating an internal pouch from the small intestine to collect the waste material.

It was hard listening after option number two. I was numb: never having heard of people living without a colon, I was getting more convinced I didn't want any of that.

Dr. W asked if I understood everything he said, which forced me to refocus, and I nodded, signaling yes. "Normally I tell patients that they have time to make a decision," he continued, "but your case does not give us plenty of time. You have to decide as soon as possible before your condition worsens. As far as my part, I will make myself available when you decide to move, immediately." He continued to explain all three surgical options ran the risk of my losing my ability to achieve an erection. "In that case you can use medications such as Viagra," he said, "and you may not be able to ejaculate, but you will be able to experience orgasm, only it will be dry."

I was very ambivalent about the surgery up to this point, but now I became increasingly convinced that the risk was too great. My thoughts were that I'm not going this route, no matter what the consequences. After my previous two surgeries, resuming sexual activity took no longer than two to three weeks post-hospitalization. This time I learned the challenges I would face would be much greater.

I'd started reconsidering the tapes I'd watched of Dr. Day's nonsurgical methods. They suddenly looked more attractive. Then I remembered that Dr. W used to work at UCSF in the same hospital as Dr. Day, so I asked him if he knew her. He did, but he was unaware of her changing camps and completely disapproving of conventional treatments for cancer. All he remembered was that she had been an activist, organizing doctors to protect themselves from contracting AIDS while treating patient who were HIV positive. The other thing he knew about her was that her spouse was also a doctor. I couldn't get any comment from him regarding her methods.

I then asked Dr. W if it were possible to reverse my cancer using natural methods. His answer surprised me: he'd once had a patient who was diagnosed with Stage IV cancer, meaning it had spread to her liver and he couldn't help her. That woman went home and started drinking fruit and vegetable juices every hour or so, and when she came back after a year for a checkup, her cancer was gone. Dr. W said he couldn't explain or understand it, and he couldn't recommend it as a treatment.

My case was not hopeless, and the option of drinking juices as a treatment carried a very high risk of the cancer spreading to other organs. Dr. W also told me that a colectomy, proctectomy, and ileostomy (option number one) was very rare in colon cancer cases and was usually only necessary for people who have been diagnosed with inflammatory bowel disease, also known as Crohn's disease. Most patients who received such surgery would consider their quality of life to be greatly improved compared with how they had felt before. However, because I'd had no previous problems and had only Stage II cancer, rather than being improved, my quality of life would likely deteriorate after such procedures, and the psychological aspect of this surgery could have an impact.

Dr. W spent more than an hour explaining all the options available to me. He was very patient, answered all my questions, and gave us time to think it over. Before he sent us to the stoma nurse, he called in Dr. F, the oncologist who had participated in the tumor board discussion. Dr. F was familiar with my situation and gave us an overview of the treatment I might need after surgery. He recommended starting with adjuvant chemotherapy treatment a few weeks later after I'd regained my strength. "You've had two recurrences, and we have to make sure no cancer cells remain in your body." I couldn't help but think that was exactly what Dr. H had recommended after the first surgery. I should have listened to him, but now it was too late—I needed to deal with the present situation rather than focusing on what I could have done.

The next stop was a visit with the stoma nurse. I didn't know what a stoma nurse does, and at that point I didn't care. Emotionally, I was in a state of confusion—the whole thing seemed like a bad dream. I was planning my funeral in my head, my prognosis looked very bleak … then I heard my name being called.

The stoma nurse led us to a back room and asked me to take my upper body clothes off and sit down. She explained that her job was to take care of the new opening I would have on my abdomen—sort of my new rectum. The reason I needed to see her before surgery was to mark the exact spot where the opening should be.

For the surgeon, she made a circle above where the body folds in a seated position. She then trained me how to empty the bag when it gets one-third full by sitting at the very back of the toilet seat and releasing the clip, then using toilet paper to clean it up.

I heard her, but nothing sank in; it was like she was talking to me from a distance. None of this applied to me, I thought—I wasn't going to need any of that anyway, so this talk was just a waste of time.

She ended with giving me printed literature with support group phone numbers and a description of the stoma system. Before we left, she also mentioned a few names of famous people who were living with ostomies, including one golf champion; however by the time we were out of there, I couldn't remember any of them, and I made no effort to call any of the support groups. This was a mistake, as I let my emotions take over my thinking. Today I play an active role in a support group, and more then once I've met people who come to the meeting before having the surgery. This prepares them better for the challenges they will face afterwards.

We were outside of the hospital, talking on the sidewalk, when I told Shoshi and Yaniv that I wasn't going to go through this: the cancer had returned, and I didn't see any point in doing the same thing that hadn't worked twice in the past. Shoshi was very emotional, fighting her tears and demanding that without wasting any time, we go back to schedule surgery with Dr. W. Yaniv also agreed the surgery was the best option we had.

We sat down on a bench in front of the hospital, and for the next hour or more, Yaniv and Shoshi tried to persuade me to schedule the surgery because time was of the essence. I kept repeating that I didn't want to become a useless body that would need to be supported by an outside system I didn't yet understand. It was a very emotional discussion; Shoshi, in tears, was saying that she refused to be alone, and I kept repeating that useless body claim.

I was very troubled with my decision, as I wasn't sure if I had the moral right to make a decision by myself that would affect my entire family, especially my loving wife. I thought about the young widows I knew, and I was getting close to the breaking point. I didn't want to die, of course, but at that moment, the idea of being dependent and a burden to my family, especially my wife, looked much worse than dying.

I shared my moral dilemma with Yaniv, whose view was that morally I had the right to do as I wish, because, as he put it, we all arrive and leave this world alone—he only questioned the wisdom of this choice. Eventually we went home without making any decision as I needed more time to digest my situation.

When we got home, the first thing I did was call Dr. H to hear an unemotional, professional point of view regarding my treatment options. His wife answered the call, and in her usual nice and supportive way promised that Dr. H would call as soon as he got home from the clinic. When he did so a few hours later, he did a very good job of lifting my spirits. There was no reason to panic, he said. Yes, living with a bag as a colon replacement wasn't pleasant, but it wasn't the end of the world either. He had a number of patients with ostomy bags, and they all were doing fine. You can learn to live with it, he said, and considering the alternative, it was not so bad. Dr. H thought that if I did nothing, I would be dead within a year.

As far as the three options, he recommended the first one—the complete removal of the colon and the rectum, having an ostomy bag. "If you choose any other option, you might as well tell them to make you a zipper on your abdomen for easy removal of infected body parts in the future so they can avoid the need to cut you up again," he said. I got the point, but what about sexual side effects? Yes these risks are real, he said, but I was in good hands. "Stanford is a renowned institution, and as you told me, your surgeon did a good job twice already, so have confidence in him." I didn't know how to thank my friend; he had spent hours talking with me and reading my medical records since I was first diagnosed without expecting anything in return. I felt very lucky to have him as my unbiased expert.

At this point I started rethinking my objection to surgery. Maybe I was making a second mistake, and this time my life was on the line. That night I went to sleep uneasy and not exactly sure what to do.

In the morning while having breakfast, Shoshi, Yaniv, and I discussed the situation again, trying to agree on a strategy. Shoshi kept pressuring me to make an appointment for surgery without losing any more time. She was worried the cancer would spread, and she demanded quick action. The idea came up to call Dr. L, my GI specialist. But I wasn't ready yet to accept the fact that another surgery was inevitable. I wasted a few more days watching Dr. Day's tapes once more before I picked up the phone to call Dr. L. I knew that if I called his office, I would be subjected to the normal questioning, and it was very unlikely I would be able to reach him. I decided instead to use the pager number he'd given me. Within a few minutes after my call, the phone rang. I didn't think it was Dr. L calling back so soon, but there he was.

I thanked him for responding so quickly and told him about the options I remembered Dr. W presenting, adding that I was debating between doing nothing and the second option of connecting the small intestine to the rectum—at least on the outside I would be the same. Dr. L then spent the next half hour persuading me that I'd chosen the two worst options. "You are married, have grown children, and you are over fifty years old," he said. "You want the best odds to be in your favor. It's like going to Vegas—don't you want to have the best odds when gambling there?"

He then said something that really resonated with me: "You're not a cat with nine lives … you've already been given three … don't risk the fourth. You have only one option, and it is option number one." In other words, I needed to get rid of my troublemaking organs.

When I got off the phone, I took a moment to reflect: yes, I had cancer, but I never at any point felt anger or self-pity. I also didn't necessarily feel lucky, although if I hadn't been exercising regularly, I probably wouldn't have detected the problem in time. And as for treatment needed, I *was* very lucky to have the best possible team on my side. Not only were they experts in their fields, they also really cared. I decided to keep fighting—the combination of a loving, supportive family and a top-of-the-line professional team was a winning one, and I had to do my part. The next day, I called to schedule the surgery.

15
The Third Surgery

I was asked to go to the Stanford Clinic for a series of tests before surgery could be scheduled. On September 16th, I had blood work performed, two days later I delivered stool samples to the Stanford lab, and the next day I had my first positron emission tomography (PET) scan. This test is similar to a CT scan in that they inject radioactive material through an IV that produces an image of the internal organs. On the 22nd, I met the anesthesiologist and had an electrocardiogram (ECG). The PET scan did not detect any spread of the cancer to other organs (the liver was of special concern). However, the blood tests showed I was still anemic, and the stool test was positive for blood. Nothing had changed miraculously. I was ready for my biggest fight yet. Surgery was scheduled for Monday, September 26, 2005. I asked to be the first patient, and again my wish was granted.

As my blood level was low, we were told a blood transfusion might be necessary during surgery, and we were given the option of having a family member donate. Shoshi and Yaniv agreed so I could avoid the small risk of getting contaminated blood—one less thing to worry about. We got the address of the blood bank, which was within walking distance of the hospital, and we registered at the window. The line was long, and it took an hour for our names to be called.

Shoshi was first. She followed the nurse to the station chair where she was given a form to complete regarding her health history. After she passed this step successfully, she was given a long list of countries and asked if she'd visited any of them during the past year. If so, she was disqualified from donating blood. There were three countries on the list we'd all visited during the past year (Japan, Thailand, and Cambodia), so neither Shoshi nor Yaniv's blood could be accepted. Avi offered to come down and give blood, but the late hour and the need for two units made this idea unfeasible. I was disappointed, but optimistic that blood would not be needed; after all, I'd already had two surgeries without requiring a transfusion, so there was no reason to believe this time would be any different.

We arrived at the hospital a little after 6:30 a.m. I registered at the appropriate window and sat down to wait for my name to be called. I saw Dr. W walking down the hall and was surprised that he started so early, as even if I were called right away, it would take another hour before I was completely prepared for surgery. The circle on my abdomen that was marked for the opening by the stoma nurse had begun to fade. I suppose it wasn't meant to last more than a couple of days, and I worried the ostomy would be placed in the wrong spot. In case I forgot, I asked Shoshi to mention this to the operating team before they took me in.

My name was called, and I walked straight to the preparation room. Shortly afterwards I was lying down on the hospital bed wearing only the gown and answering all the standard questions before surgery the nurse had on the form. The anesthesiologist started an IV and then asked for my preferred method. Again I requested there be no epidural, which was noted on the form.

The next step was for me to sign the consent form. The procedure described on the form was: a complete proctocolectomy with end ileostomy. The only word I recognized was *complete*, which I translated as meaning a complete removal of the colon. I asked the nurse to confirm it, and after she did I signed the form with a shaky hand. I knew that when I woke up, I would not be the same inside anymore. I always wonder why the medical profession insists on communicating with us in a lingo they know we don't understand, especially when they ask us for our consent for a risky treatment.

Before they rolled the bed to surgery, Dr. W came to check me, and I used the opportunity to mention the fading mark. He said not to worry, that everything would be fine. His confident voice was the last thing I remembered before I fell into a deep sleep.

The first thing I saw when I woke up was Shoshi's loving and worried face. She told me that the surgery had taken more than five-and-a-half hours, a lot longer than the previous two. I felt very weak and fell asleep again. The first twenty-four hours after surgery I spent mostly sleeping; I finally woke up in the middle of the night to find a nurse taking my vitals (meaning temperature, blood pressure, and pulse). My room door was open, and the number read E 323A. Shoshi was sleeping on a bed next to me that had been provided by the staff.

The nurse asked if I felt any pain, and when I nodded yes, she instructed me on how to use the morphine button, which automatically delivered morphine through the IV. After the first two surgeries I'd seldom used it, but this time the pain level was much higher and the button became very useful.

Early in the morning the light was turned on, and a lab person came to take blood samples. Half an hour later the doctors came for the morning rounds. They looked at the incision and encouraged me to use the pain button for relief. I asked the lead doctor if I was given any blood during surgery; the answer was negative, but I was not out of the woods yet. He told me that because my blood level was still low, Dr. W would make the decision on that.

Two days after surgery I got up for the first time, but I couldn't walk more than a few steps. Pain was a major problem, and the morphine button was a close friend. Dr. W came to visit, and although he gave me a good report on the surgery in general, he said I had lost too much blood. He'd hoped my body would start replacing the lost blood, but as it was doing it too slowly, he ordered two units of blood for me.

Later that day when the nurse walked in with two units of blood, I wanted to make sure that it was my blood type—O positive—before it was hooked up to the IV. I believe that as a patient I have the responsibility of being actively involved in my treatment if I can, which means knowing the medications I get (including their dosage and frequency) so as to help the hospital staff prevent mistakes. The Stanford Hospital staff was really wonderful, providing top-level care. However, I knew how hard they worked to look after so many patients, and I was certain they appreciated any help they could get. Shoshi was thanked many times for her willingness to assume the simple responsibilities of emptying the ostomy bag, helping me wash myself, and so on. It freed the staff to care for other patients who had less family support. And for me, her loving care was a crucial factor in my recovery.

For the first week I could not look at my ostomy. Shoshi emptied it most of the time, and during the night I rang the nurse to let Shoshi sleep. Only after I was discharged from the hospital did I dare to look at it. I tried to take longer walks every day, but eating was a problem. I didn't have any appetite and nothing looked good, so I kept losing weight. A nutrition expert was sent to advise me on what to eat. I expected to hear from her that I needed to increase my intake of healthy foods such as fruits and vegetables, but she asked if I liked ice cream. "You need to gain weight," she explained, "so don't hesitate to request items like ice cream and cake when you order food from the menu." Yet I had no desire for any of that. I tried to think about all my favorite foods, but I couldn't come up with anything appealing.

Another challenge I faced was with breathing. Every so often, I would forget to breathe. I was told this was a result of the drugs used for anesthesia. Shoshi and the children were always on guard to make sure I was breathing.

On the third day after surgery, the stoma nurse came for the first time. I remembered her as she was the one who'd marked the exit spot on my abdomen for the surgeon. She commented that my stoma looked very nice and complimented the surgeon on a job well done. Then she wanted to teach me how to use the ostomy bag, but it was way too soon for me: I had not yet accepted my new situation.

Shoshi volunteered to be trained instead. The stoma nurse came every other day with a toolbox filled with all the spare parts and different sizes and shapes of accessories, and she watched while Shoshi changed the bag. Shoshi learned the job very quickly, and I was very comfortable having her change the bag for me, but I knew this was my job and I would have to learn how to do it soon.

My recovery continued at a slow pace, with my next goal being to have the catheter removed. This depended very much on my urine output, so I tried to drink as much as I could, but it was not enough. On the one hand, I wasn't producing adequate amounts of urine, but on the other, my bag output was excessive. I was always careful to make sure the nurse recorded my urine output on the chart, even if it was only a few drops. My bag had the opposite problem: it was overly active, which had to be controlled because it was causing dehydration.

Dr. W prescribed Lomotil to control the output. I had to take two pills three times a day under the tongue.

My walks were getting longer every day, and when the IV was disconnected, we started leaving the hospital building. I enjoyed the sun's warmth sitting with Shoshi by the fountain. Many friends came to visit and offer their support, and there were other kinds of visitors as well. Our own rabbi came often; a local rabbi came every Friday to pray with us; a priest came and read from the Bible; and a number of volunteers stopped by. Those visits were always uplifting and a morale boost for both of us. I made sure to remember their names and ask about their lives. One volunteer was getting married in the coming months, and he was very excited about the wedding that would take place in South America, his bride's home country. Another came from Switzerland and enjoyed spending some of her time visiting hospital patients.

Two weeks went by, and my condition hadn't changed much. My weight kept falling, my urine output was still low, and my bag output was still too high. The only bright side was the walks. They were getting longer and longer, and I spent more time outdoors.

Every day blood was taken for testing, and even though I'd received two units, blood count improvement was very slow to the point that I started wondering if the tumor was still present. Another challenge was urinating, but despite the low output, a decision was made that the catheter would be removed the next day. Afterwards I made a conscious effort to drink as much as possible, but my difficulties with urinating persisted. The medical team ordered a CT scan so they could determine the source of the problem. A bottle of white liquid was delivered to my room for me to drink so as to give a good contrast to the CT images. It took me a while to finish the awful-tasting stuff.

Then I waited for the transport team to take me to the first floor so the scan could be performed. After two hours went by with no one appearing, I started getting edgy. I knew there was a time limit on the effectiveness of the contrast liquid, and I really didn't want to drink it again. Shoshi kept going to the nurses' station, but it was out of their control. The ball was in the court of the Radiology Department. The nurse brought to our attention the frequent trips of the helicopter ambulance that was visible from my room and the possibility that many emergencies were backing up Radiology.

Six hours later, I was still struggling to urinate, so Shoshi returned to the nurses' station to inquire about the status of the scan. They agreed to call Radiology, only to find out that the CT scan order had been misplaced. As I expected, when we finally got to Radiology, I had to drink the contrast medication once more. I was very frustrated at that point but didn't have a choice. I drank it again slowly, fighting the urge to throw up.

The CT scan didn't reveal anything unusual, and the next test ordered was an ultrasound to see if my bladder was full or empty. Demand for the portable ultrasound machine apparently was very high that day, and my pain due to the inability to urinate was increasing by the minute to the point a doctor had to be paged. When the shift doctor came, he immediately ordered a new catheter. As soon as it was in, the bag filled with urine and I was relieved. The ultrasound test was canceled as my bladder was obviously full. This was my first setback since the surgery, and I was disappointed.

The next day, Dr. W asked us to closely monitor the urine output; if no improvement were achieved, he would ask a urologist to examine me. The ostomy bag output did not change and continued to be excessive. The Lomotil pills had not made any difference yet, and it was mentioned that if there were no positive results soon from the Lomotil, the next step would be opium. This was a scary thought for me: all I needed now was to get hooked on street drugs! I didn't know this at the time, but medical opium is not addictive. I decided that if it were offered, I'd refuse to take it. This was quite premature on my part.

However, I have since learned why they were hesitant to give me opium: it was the strongest drug in the arsenal to fight diarrhea, and it was not a good idea to use this weapon until all other options were exhausted. In the following days, a slight improvement was recorded in both areas—the urine output was increasing and iliostomy output was decreasing. I felt a little stronger even though my weight loss continued. The Lomotil dose was reduced to twice a day, and I started seeing myself leaving the hospital soon. This was important to me because the long stay was taking a toll on Shoshi. She was sleeping only a few hours at night on a very uncomfortable bed and her back was bothering her, but she never once complained. Her focus was totally on me and my recovery.

The next blood test indicated an improvement in blood count, and I became more optimistic about going home soon. The next day when Dr. W came to examine me, he seemed somewhat satisfied with my overall condition, but the excessive output of the ostomy and low urine volume still concerned him. On October 14th, three weeks after my surgery, a large group of doctors came to evaluate me. They spent a long time discussing my situation and reading all the reports, and they eventually decided to discharge me if I could urinate on my own.

After the doctors left, the head nurse came in to inform us of a test she would perform shortly. She would inject 400 cc of water through the catheter directly into my bladder, and then remove the catheter. My task was to urinate all 400 cc within a few minutes. If successful, I would be discharged that day. It was very exciting news for me: I was looking forward to continuing my recovery at home, and I was already visualizing myself lounging in our sunny backyard reading and listening to my favorite classical music.

Around noontime when my lunch was brought, the nurse came in, waited until I was finished eating, then injected the water through the catheter and immediately removed it. I was so nervous and uptight that I was afraid it would prevent me from urinating. I tried to relax, and within minutes I felt the urge to urinate. I came very close to the 400 cc required—this was my ticket out! All that was left now was for Dr. W to sign the discharge paperwork and we could go home. Shoshi called Avi with the exciting news that we needed a ride home, and he was happy to come pick us up.

When we arrived home, we had a surprise waiting for us: Orit and Avi had painted our living room. Shoshi had talked about her desire to do it for quite some time now, and they had finally made it happen. Orit had also prepared the downstairs room for me so I wouldn't have to climb the stairs to our bedroom on the second floor until I regained my strength.

16
Home Sweet Home

Returning home after being away on vacation was always a good feeling to me. Even though I enjoyed my vacation, my own home, my own bed, and my familiar surroundings gave me joy. Returning home after a hospital stay was a thousand times sweeter. Although I still struggled with simple tasks such as walking and eating, I was very happy to be home. I was prescribed Vicodin for pain relief and prochlorperazine for nausea and vomiting and given a phone number if something went wrong, such as liquids on the incision wound.

Shoshi was still changing the bag for me, but the time had come for me to be trained how to do it by myself. The iliostomy output didn't show any sign of reduction, and I was having a problem drinking enough water to keep myself from dehydrating. I spent most of my days watching television or reading as well as enjoying the time with friends when they came to visit.

Five days after discharge, I noticed the iliostomy output was drastically reduced. At first I was happy the Lomotil had finally started working. But soon after, I started having severe abdominal pain, and the iliostomy output completely stopped. The day I was discharged I'd been given a list of foods to avoid (corn, lettuce, spinach, and other kinds of leafy greens) because they could cause a blockage. I was careful not to eat any of these foods, but apparently something was blocking my system.

When the pain became unbearable and I started vomiting, Shoshi called the phone number I'd been given. After she described my symptoms, we were ordered to come to Stanford Hospital's Emergency Room (ER) immediately. After we arrived and I completed all the tests, my medical team was notified and they all came down to examine me. I was given medication for the pain and sent to Radiology for an enema to open the blockage. I was wondering how exactly they would give me one as I didn't have a rectum. The doctor read my mind and explained they would enter through the ostomy.

But when we arrived at Radiology, the technician who was supposed to perform the enema had left early, and no one else could do the job. After a short consultation with Dr. W over the phone, they decided to keep me overnight and do the enema in the morning. The nurse started an IV and then transported me to the same department I'd left only five days ago. The staff expressed their surprise to see me back and did all they could to make me feel comfortable. The pain medication started having an effect, and I soon fell asleep. Shoshi tried to sleep on a chair next to me, but it wasn't easy—any sign of pain from me would cause her to jump, and the light turning on every time a nurse came to take my vitals was disturbing to her.

When I woke up, it was almost morning, and I no longer felt any pain. At first I thought the pain medication I'd received must have been very strong, but then I noticed my bag was totally full and about to burst any second. I frantically asked Shoshi to empty it for me. When the doctors' team came for their morning rounds, I was feeling much better, and as there was no longer a need for the enema, I was sent home armed with pain relief pills and a list of foods that were okay to eat. Apparently, whatever was blocking the ostomy had worked its way out by itself.

We returned home in the early afternoon on Thursday, October 20th. I was hoping for some quiet time, but it was not to be. The ostomy was working overtime and needed to be emptied every hour or so. It seemed that my system had only two speeds, stop and overdrive, neither of which was good for me.

On top of it all, I again started having difficulty urinating. By Saturday this problem had gotten worse. I told Shoshi I probably would need a catheter to help me urinate, but it was a weekend and I didn't want to go to the ER again. The problem persisted, and Shoshi decided to call Dr. S, my physician, to ask for advice. She left a message on the home answering machine (we are members at the same temple), and he called back shortly afterwards. He prescribed Flomax and called it in to the Walgreens pharmacy for us to pick up. He also recommended I come to the clinic on Monday morning for a checkup.

I remembered I'd been getting Flomax in the hospital once a day. Shoshi asked a friend to pick up the medication from the pharmacy as she didn't want to leave me alone. When I received it, I started taking it immediately. However, the expected relief didn't materialize. Maybe just more time was needed, but now I was really looking forward to Monday morning when I would get the catheter inserted and be relieved.

On Monday morning, Shoshi and I were the first people in the office, and soon I was sitting on the examination bed. Dr. S pressed on my abdomen around the bladder area. As he didn't feel anything in my bladder, he concluded I didn't need a catheter and instead referred me to a urologist. The office manager placed the call to a local urology clinic and arranged for me to have an appointment within an hour.

We drove to the clinic, which was about fifteen minutes away, and after a short wait we were led to the exam room. I was asked by the nurse to urinate into a cup. Very little came out, but it was enough for the urine test. When the urologist came in, he said that no blood was found in my urine, and he hooked me up to an ultrasound machine. The ultrasound revealed that my bladder was completely empty. "How can you expect to urinate if you don't drink?" he asked. "Go to the waiting room and drink ten glasses of water from the water stand, and tell the nurse when you need to go." It didn't take too long before that came about. Apparently I wasn't drinking enough and had just panicked when I couldn't urinate. It was a big relief to know that my prostate was not the problem.

The urologist wanted to know about my future treatments. I told him about the chemotherapy I would have to start soon. He mentioned I had the option of doing it locally; he said there was no need to drive all the way to Stanford, as they did it where we were just as well. "I'm sure you do," I replied, "but I'm already used to the Stanford system, and I'm very happy with them." He then asked me to come again in three months for a checkup. We thanked him and drove home with a big sense of relief. My problem was only imaginary, not real.

From that point on, in preparation for the chemotherapy I dreaded so much, I made sure to remember to drink just about every hour and also eat more so I could regain some of the weight I'd lost. The ostomy output didn't improve much, so I started experimenting with food. Rice and potatoes had a reputation for causing constipation, but they didn't work for me. I tried bananas, which were also no help. One evening Shoshi asked if I cared for some chestnuts that she'd bought from the local market. She knew that I loved chestnuts, and

I enthusiastically said yes. And as I usually do, I overate. Besides the rich flavor of the chestnuts there was an added benefit: my ostomy finally began to slow down. We added chestnuts to our dinner menu as the dessert.

17
The Aftermath

October 27, 2005, was the date of my first appointment with Dr. F at Stanford's Oncology Clinic. This was the step I had refused to take twice in the past because of fear of side effects from chemotherapy. My friend Dr. H had done all he could to persuade me of the necessity of the treatment, but to no avail. At this point it was clear to me I should have had chemo after the first surgery, but that opportunity was lost. Now my focus was on getting the benefits from the chemo with as little damage as possible.

Dr. F, a very nice man with a calming smile whom I had first met after the tumor board meeting two months earlier, made me feel comfortable with the first handshake. "We did not think you needed chemotherapy at first," he said, "but with two recurrences of the cancer, we now recommend six cycles of chemotherapy treatments for the next six months." He continued to explain that I would have to come to the fusion clinic after giving blood at the lab and seeing him for evaluation. At the fusion clinic, I would receive oxaliplatin through an IV; this would be essentially a day-long event. Then for the following two weeks, I would take Xeloda at home twice a day: five pills in the morning and four in the evening. As Dr. F explained to me, Xeloda, also known as 5-FU, is the first oral chemotherapy treatment available for colon cancer; oxaliplatin was approved not long ago. This was a combination of pills and IV treatment. Then I got one week off before the cycle began again—a day for IV treatment and two weeks of pills—for a total of six cycles.

The side effects from the treatment could include one or all of the following: tingling of the fingertips and toes; sensitivity to cold; a strange feeling in the throat; inability to eat any cold or solid foods (only smooth foods such as broth, jelly, and pudding were recommended); bleeding easily, which would be hard to stop during shaving or use of other sharp objects; a high risk of infection; fatigue; and feeling sleepy. I would need to keep my mouth and teeth very clean and moist, to use nonabrasive toothpaste, and to be careful using dental floss because the mouth is a very sensitive area when blood counts are at the lowest level from the chemo. Dr. F added another thing to be aware of was a weakened immune system; during chemo, some degree of isolation might be a good idea to minimize the risk of infection. I had plenty of information to digest before my first chemo cycle, which was scheduled for November 3rd. At this point I'd already accepted that my philosophy about medication would have to be suspended for at least the duration of the chemotherapy, but I was still very fearful of the side effects.

On Thursday morning at 9:00 a.m., Shoshi and I arrived at the Oncology Clinic for the first cycle of the chemo treatment. I was a little apprehensive—fear of the unknown is always a challenge to overcome, and I had no idea what to expect. After the blood work was completed, Dr. F conducted a general exam, and then we were sent to the fusion center upstairs for the treatment. It had about six rooms, with every room having eight reclining chairs with a TV screen and IV stand adjacent. In front of the rooms was a long corridor with nurses' stations. We were led to the third room by Nurse E, and I got a chair with a view (I was told this was because it was my first time). All the chairs were taken, and many more patients awaited their turn. I looked around and saw mostly young people: men and women, some with no hair, many with masks, hooked up to IVs. I looked at their faces and read sadness, apathy, and fear. I looked for a mirror to see what my face was projecting, and it was no different. This was a very depressing environment.

Nurse E told us that someone would be with me shortly to start an IV, and she checked the paperwork to make sure I was the right guy. Another nurse came and tried to get the IV going with no luck. After she made a few holes in both of my arms, she gave up, apologized, and went to get help. Another nurse came—I assumed a more experienced one—and managed to start an IV on the back of my hand where the most visible vein was found. I was given a handful of pills to take before treatment began in order to prevent nausea and vomiting.

By the time the chemo started flowing, I felt indifferent to my surroundings. I slept on and off. Shoshi was reading, and the time passed very slowly. I'd been told the process usually takes about four to five hours, but by the second hour, my hand had started to swell. At first it didn't hurt, but as time went by, I started feeling pain. I showed my hand to Shoshi, and she went looking for the nurse. The nurses were very busy hooking and unhooking patients and it took some time to get their attention. Eventually one came, looked at my hand, and said she didn't see anything wrong.

Half an hour later the pain got worse, and we called for help again. A different nurse came, and as soon as she saw my hand, she started moving very fast. "Why didn't you say anything?" she yelled and went to get help. I said I did, but she didn't hear me. She came back with another nurse and they disconnected the IV, which apparently had not been administered correctly, thus causing the swelling. She then looked at my left hand for a good vein to use. It took some time, but she found one, and from that point forward the process went smoothly.

By the time it was over I was tired but didn't feel anything different. However, a few moments later when we left the building and felt the chilly outside air, I experienced the tingling feeling Dr. F had described as a possible side effect. Even putting my hands in my pockets did not help much. Shoshi had to do the driving because I couldn't touch anything.

It was late evening when we arrived home and sat down to eat dinner. Shoshi made a delicious soup, and I ate it warm. I decided then I would start the chemo pills, Xeloda, the next morning after breakfast.

As soon as I started to take the pills, my condition began deteriorating by the day. I was eating very little and couldn't go anywhere, even to the backyard, as I had to stay indoors all the time. On top of that, I was hit with severe diarrhea. I had to empty the bag every forty-five minutes or so, and the contents were 90 percent water. I couldn't even drink tap water—it was too cold for me—so I had to warm the water before drinking, and it was a constant battle to drink enough to match the liquids I was losing—an impossible mission. I felt like I was taking poison twice a day, and I had to keep reminding myself that I had to do it to save my life.

My condition continued to deteriorate: walking became difficult, visits to the bathroom were frequent, and eating was almost impossible. Shoshi offered me all my favorite foods, but nothing was appealing. I also had a sharp abdominal pain that kept getting worse.

On the second week of the treatment, one day before finishing the pills, I could no longer tolerate it. On Thursday, November 17th, I asked Shoshi to call the Oncology Clinic for advice. After describing my condition, we were asked to come to the clinic right away.

We arrived at the clinic around noon and headed straight for the second floor. I could barely walk up the stairs, and only when I was halfway there did I realize I should have taken the elevator. We were taken to the treatment room immediately, and the attending doctor was called because Dr. F was out. The attending doctor ordered a blood test and an IV, and the nurse came to do both at the same time so I would be poked only once. This was the first time I saw my blood so dark—it was almost black. When I asked about it, the nurse said it was because I was severely dehydrated. She did all she could to make me feel comfortable, bringing blankets, offering beverages, and being very nice to us.

After being on the IV for two hours, I felt a little better, but the abdominal pain remained. After a few more hours of fluids, I was able to walk to the bathroom a lot easier; soon thereafter the IV was removed and I was sent to Radiology for abdominal and chest X-rays. When the results came back, something was not right, and the doctor decided to keep me overnight for observation. This was called a twenty-three-hour observation and was different from hospitalization, which was more than a twenty-four-hour stay. The reason it was done that way was to save me the trouble of going through the ER—a very unpleasant experience.

Back in the room, a different doctor ordered more tests. I gave more blood, and urine and stool samples were sent to the lab. During the night Shoshi had to empty the ostomy bag almost every hour or less. Needless to say, neither of us slept much.

In the morning I felt a little better, but the abdominal pain was still there. The lab results showed some blood in the urine. That was a new finding, another thing to worry about. When the doctors made their rounds, I overheard them talking about me. They weren't so sure what to do with me—keep me longer or send me home? So they asked me if I felt well enough to go home. I didn't want to stay, so I told them I felt better, if not completely well. Within an hour the discharge order came along with instructions for me to follow up with my physician on the blood-in-the-urine problem. I also needed to confirm my appointment with Dr. F in two weeks for the second cycle of chemo, and the order recommended that Dr. F consider reducing the dose of Xeloda, the chemo pills. We went home, although both of us felt that maybe I should have stayed in the hospital.

I was told not to take the remaining pills until I saw Dr. F. My diarrhea did not show any sign of letting up and the abdominal pain started worsening again, so the day after my discharge, I asked Shoshi to call the Oncology Clinic and try to reach Dr. F. She left a message, and someone called back in the afternoon. Shoshi described my situation, and we were told to come to the ER.

On the way to the hospital, I asked Shoshi to go first to the Oncology Clinic as maybe we could skip the ER. She didn't think this was a good idea, but I insisted—after all, I'd just gotten discharged. It didn't work: they put me in a wheelchair and rolled me to the ER.

It was not a good day to be in the ER: a Stanford football game had just ended and the ER was filled with intoxicated spectators and tailgaters. The staff had their hands full trying to take care of all the patients, and it took me more than an hour just to be checked in, followed by a long wait in the hallway for a free spot. A nurse tried to start an IV, but before finishing had to leave for other emergencies. Finally, after I'd waited a few hours, the IV was started and the attending doctor came to examine me. While the nurse was checking my temperature and blood pressure, the doctor asked many questions and wrote down my answers on a clipboard. I tried to describe the last eighteen months in a few minutes, and then the doctor left to call Dr. W or one of his aides. Some time later an ECG machine was brought in, and the technician started to hook me up to it. I tried to tell him that my heart was fine, but he had his orders to perform the test. The doctor came back, telling us that he had talked to my medical team and I would need a CT scan to determine the source of the abdominal pain.

While I was waiting for my turn for the CT scan, we witnessed many dramas going on all around us. To my left a drunken woman was arguing with the police officer who'd brought her in; she refused to give any personal information and denied she'd had anything to drink. An older man was having a heart attack. More police officers came in with a woman arrested in a local coffee shop for overdosing on drugs. She was yelling that all she'd had was coffee, but to no effect. Football game spectators kept coming, and at times it was hard to tell what there were more of, police officers or medical staff.

I had to make a few trips to the bathroom, dragging the IV stand with me, before my name was called to the CT room. The nurse had to change the IV for a bigger size, and it didn't go well. She went to get help. I was left alone for about fifteen minutes shivering until another nurse came to get the IV going. She struggled with it for a while and eventually succeeded in getting it in a vein. The iodine started flowing through my body, and I felt the familiar, warm feeling in my chest. The machine started talking while I was sliding into the tunnel. "Hold your breath—breathe in," I was told, and a few moments later it was done and I was sent back to my corner.

It took some time for the images to be ready. They revealed the presence of abdominal fluids. I was admitted to the hospital for interventional radiology, or as they noted it on the admission form, drainage of the fluid collection. In other words, they needed to get the fluid out somehow. By the time a room was found for me, it was late at night and I was exhausted. The night shift nurse tried to find a bed for Shoshi, but nothing was available. She had to sleep in a chair next to me, which was not good for her back, but she refused to go home.

In the morning I was taken to Radiology, and a hose was inserted through my abdomen. A CT scan helped guide the hose to the right spot by the pelvis for drainage of the fluid. When I returned to the room, another bag hung from my left side to collect fluids—mainly blood left there during the surgery. The biology report came back negative for bacterial growth, but nevertheless I was treated with IV antibiotics. After two days the IV was removed, which made walking easier, so my walks became longer and longer.

On the fourth day, Dr. W came in, sat on my bed, and said, "I don't think we're doing anything good for you here; it would be better for you to go home. There isn't too much fluid coming out, your fever is down, and it seems your appetite is better." I agreed with his assessment and looked forward to going home. Some time later the nurse came and removed the drainage bag. I was discharged four days after admission, with a follow-up appointment with Dr. F on December 2nd.

By the day of my appointment I was feeling better, although the diarrhea had not stopped. The one-week break I'd had from chemo helped me gain some weight, and most of the side effects were gone. Dr. F looked at the blood test results and said they also looked good, but he decided to give me two more weeks off chemo so I could gain more strength before my second cycle. He also reduced the Xeloda dose to three pills in the morning and two in the evening. I was happy with his decision.

On my next appointment for cycle number two, I asked for a urine test (as recommended by Dr. H) to see if traces of blood were still present in my urine. The blood test indicated my electrolytes were low, so Dr. F added magnesium and calcium separately through the IV before and after the oxaliplatin was administered. By the time I finished with the chemo, the urine test report was on the computer. The nurse told me that it still showed traces of blood, which was blamed on the diarrhea. I asked for copies of the reports, and when we returned home, I faxed them to Dr. H, followed by a phone call giving him a report on my condition, including the urine test results. While I was in the hospital, he'd tried to reach me at home and became worried when I didn't answer, so I now had his pager number in case of emergency. Dr. H agreed it was possible to have blood in the urine in extreme cases of dehydration.

I started wearing gloves to lessen the effect of the tingling of my hands. This was helpful when I needed to hold objects such as silverware or a glass of water. The smaller dose of the Xeloda pills made them easier to tolerate, but none of the side effects were eliminated, especially the diarrhea, which had gotten worse. I tried to drink warm water as much as possible, but the feeling in my throat—like I had a fish bone stuck there—made drinking very difficult. During every trip to Stanford, about an hour's drive from our home, I had to make three stops for bathroom visits each way, and more during treatment.

The third cycle started the same way, with a handful of pills to prevent nausea and vomiting, the fluids for hydration, and then the oxaliplatin with magnesium and calcium. However, this time potassium was added to the mix, which resulted in extreme pain in the hand where the IV was located. The staff was aware of the fact that potassium caused pain and suggested I ask to get it in pill form for the next cycle. I was sent home with orders to start a regimen of Lomotil and Citrucel with the hope of decreasing the frequency of having to empty the stoma bag.

Back home I tried to maintain some level of activity, mainly walking short distances such as one or two miles. I wore gloves to protect my hands, but my face was exposed. By the time I returned to my house, my face was completely numb.

On January 25, 2006, I began cycle number four. At the nurses' station where the vital signs are taken, I stepped on the scale, and the digital reading stopped at 72.0 kg. This was the first time it had reached over 70 kg since the surgery. Considering the severe diarrhea I was still suffering from, this was very good. The chemistry readings from the blood test were within normal range. Only my alkaline phosphatase was mildly elevated compared with the pre-chemo level, indicating my liver was not functioning at 100 percent. Apparently this was another side effect from the chemo.

At the fusion center, the nurse was having problems starting the IV. After so many times of being poked on both hands for repeated blood tests and IVs for the chemo, there were not too many veins left to use. The nurse recommended a central line be put in, which is a hole surgically made in the chest and kept open for the IV. However, when I asked about the risks involved, she mentioned infection as being number one, plus the special attention needed when taking showers. I begged her to keep trying my hands; I had enough challenges already and there was no need for more, especially as I was halfway done. She was very sympathetic, threw away a couple of failed needles, and eventually was successful in starting the IV.

Everything went well for the first few hours with the IV infusion. However, it was already after 5:00 p.m. and most staff members had gone home, leaving only a skeleton crew to take care of the remaining patients who were not finished with their treatments. One nurse was in charge, and she had her hands full attending to all the treatment stations in the center. Through the window I could see that it was getting dark outside. Most of the chairs around me were empty with the patients still being treated spread along a large area—too large for one person to see everybody. I was almost done, and other than the expected problems, it was uneventful until the nurse came to check on me.

The oxaliplatin was finished, and it was time to add the potassium as the dessert on the IV menu. Only half an hour more and we would be on our way home. For the first fifteen minutes, it went as expected— painful, but not beyond my level of tolerance. But then the pain level got much worse. When the nurse walked by, I asked her to disconnect the IV as I couldn't take it any more. She decreased the speed of the dripping to alleviate some of the pain but refused to disconnect the IV, explaining that my potassium was low, which was dangerous for my heart. Low levels of potassium can cause heart problems.

That was enough to scare me for a minute, but after she was gone to attend to other patients, the pain became intolerable again; this made me get up from the chair and ask Shoshi to go look for assistance. There was no one around to help, and I was getting very impatient, attempting to disconnect the IV myself. Shoshi was making great efforts to calm me down. "Just wait for the nurse—if something goes wrong there isn't even a doctor here to help you," she said. I started walking as far as the IV leash allowed me, which took a few more minutes off the clock.

A few more drops of potassium had entered my bloodstream when I saw the nurse. I frantically called her, demanding she take the thing off immediately. When she saw my face, she removed the IV right away. "There are only five minutes left," she said. "I think it's enough." The relief was instant, and on the way home I asked Shoshi to remember to ask for potassium pills for the next time.

For the next two weeks I continued with the Xeloda twice a day as ordered, and the diarrhea continued to get worse. I "went" from ten times a day to fifteen times a day, a 50 percent increase. I was taking Lomotil to control the diarrhea, but it had no effect. I was also suffering from extreme fatigue and wasn't able to maintain any level of physical activity.

On February 16th we went to the clinic for evaluation before cycle number five. I was getting close to the end of the chemo treatment, with only two more cycles to endure. I kept telling myself the worst was over: just hang in there a little bit longer, and everything would go back to normal. The examination with Dr. F was unremarkable. My blood chemistry was stable other than increased alkaline phosphatase levels that indicated continuing liver problems due to the Xeloda pills. Dr. F agreed to my request to cut in half the electrolytes being given. That meant that to alleviate the burning pain, the magnesium and potassium would be given prior to the oxaliplatin and nothing after. Chemo cycle number five went relatively well, and we went home feeling optimistic that if there were any cancer cells left in my body, this aggressive treatment should have taken care of them.

I continued to take the Xeloda pills for the next two weeks, feeling worse by the day. The frequency of bathroom visits increased to twenty-five times a day, and I couldn't possibly drink enough water to make up for fluids lost, causing me to feel even weaker. One Sunday around 10:00 a.m., our good friends Joel and Jackie came to visit, but I was not doing well. I usually don't like to see people when I'm not at my best, but Joel and Jackie were close friends, so they came in. During their visit my situation got worse: I lost my voice, and I could barely walk. Shoshi wanted to go to the hospital, but I was hoping for improvement and really didn't want to go back there.

However when the situation hadn't improved by noon, Shoshi

called the fusion center for advice. They concluded I was suffering from severe dehydration and we needed to come in immediately. Joel and Jackie volunteered to drive us, which was very helpful because Shoshi was too stressed to drive and I wasn't capable. We took a bucket so I could empty the ostomy bag without needing to stop on the way to Stanford, and Shoshi took some extra clothes in case I would have to stay.

I was taken in without delay at the fusion center. Blood was drawn for the lab, the fluids started making their way into my bloodstream through the IV, and before too long, I felt alive again. However, the decision was made to keep me in the hospital to try to control the diarrhea. As I was still taking Lomotil that had no effect, it was time to use the ultimate weapon: opium. At this point I was ready to take anything that would stop the diarrhea, and it was ordered from the pharmacy.

The opium came in the form of syrup and tasted like medicine should. It wasn't the kind I'd feared that gets you high or addicted. I began taking it a few times a day every four hours in addition to some other things, and by the third day there was a noticeable reduction in the ostomy output. This was welcome news, and my medical staff decided that as long as there were no setbacks, they would send me home the next day.

On Wednesday morning the discharge order came, and we went home. I was taking the opium every four hours, and the diarrhea improved in both frequency and consistency; I went from twenty-five times a day to fifteen, which was still too much. The next day I experienced fatigue again and lost my voice. When Shoshi called the fusion center, they told us to come in and get IV fluids. We arrived on Thursday afternoon, and after the fluid infusion I felt better. The attending doctor concluded my problem was the diarrhea resulting from taking the Xeloda, and he ordered me to come in every day for the next three days—Friday, Saturday, and Sunday—to get IV fluids, which should have a more lasting effect. He was right: after three more days of infusions and continuous improvement on the diarrhea front from the opium, I felt a lot better.

I was scheduled for chemo cycle number six in a little more than a week, and I was worried that it would set me back again. My situation started improving on a daily basis. For the first time, the diarrhea was finally getting under control, and I had started my daily walks once again. On March 16th I had a follow-up appointment with Dr. F to decide on chemo cycle number six. My blood work looked good, and my potassium was also within normal limits.

However, when Dr. F came in the room and greeted us with the usual smile and handshake, he mentioned a recent study on chemotherapy that concluded there is no proof that six cycles of chemotherapy make any difference in the success ratio as compared to five cycles. He wrote the following on the report: "Because of the patient's adverse reaction and his questionable benefit from aggressive adjuvant therapy, we feel that he has a greater chance of adverse effect with additional therapy than he has of benefit. We will ask the patient to discontinue his final cycle of Xeloda." That meant cycle number six would be skipped! I was okay with that—I had begun to feel healthy again and didn't want to go back to the hospital.

On March 19th I was back in the clinic for a CT scan to see if the chemotherapy had been successful in preventing the cancer from metastasizing to other organs. The radiology report was negative, a fact that made me and my family very happy. However, as we all know, the battle against cancer is long and continuous, and one should always be on guard. That's why frequent blood tests would be required along with CT scans every six months. On March 21st I had a clinic visit with my surgeon, Dr. W, who informed me that the CT scan looked good. Another scan was scheduled for six months.

During the time I was going through chemotherapy, I was told of a support group that met in the clinic once a month, but I was too ill to participate. Now it was time to check it out. These group meetings were run by Dr. F's assistant, and they were not only very beneficial to me, but I believe to all participants. She is a wonderful person who facilitates these meetings after a full day of work. I was sure the entire group appreciated her efforts to bring good speakers every month for our benefit. I tried to attend most meetings as I found them very helpful.

I met other people facing similar challenges and learned there are many ways of dealing with them. Having to share my story and hearing those of others made me feel less alone. There is a sort of camaraderie among the participants, and seeing people who were five years or more postsurgery made me feel hopeful.

On August 21st I had my first six-month CT scan, and on the 30th a follow-up visit with Dr. F, who reported the CT results looked good. I was excited to see that my blood levels had returned to the level of a few years ago before I was diagnosed with colon cancer. The very next day Shoshi and I flew to Israel for a well-deserved vacation, especially for Shoshi, who'd spent days and nights by my side and was very instrumental in my recovery.

18
Clues and Warning Signs

Sometimes a major disease will give clues or warning signs before it becomes a full-blown problem. My body had provided me with a few subtle hints beginning in 2004, but unfortunately I wasn't paying attention.

Wednesday morning, February 11, 2004, started as a normal working day for Shoshi and me at the waterfront deli we'd owned for the last fifteen years. I didn't have any reason to believe anything unusual would happen that day. The weather was beautiful for February, and business was very good. Our chef, Carmen, was working as fast as she could so everything would be ready before lunchtime. Our deli was known for the quality and freshness of the food and the friendly and speedy service, in spite of the fact we were always busy. The deli was located in the beautiful Marina Village in Alameda, where the clientele consisted mainly of high-tech workers from the surrounding offices along with the boat owners and the people who served them in the marina. Carmen started work at 6:00 a.m. and began to work on the day's menu. By around 11:00 a.m., the cooking was almost completed for the day, and we were getting ready for the lunch rush when I went to the bathroom. While washing my hands, I noticed the color of the water in the sink was changing to red. It took me a few seconds to realize the red water was really blood dripping from my nose. As I attempted to stop the bleeding by blowing my nose, the dripping became a stream, and in spite all my efforts to stop it using a handful of paper towels, it was getting worse. When I lifted my head to slow the bleeding, I felt the blood in my throat. I started spitting to avoid swallowing it, and chunks of blood came out of my throat.

I ran back to the deli, and as soon as Shoshi saw me, she gave me three terry-cloth towels to replace the paper towels I was holding over my nose. I knew something was wrong and I needed to go to the hospital. I'd never had anything like that happen to me before. However, the problem was timing: it was 11:30 a.m., just before the lunch rush, and as I couldn't drive myself, someone would have to take me. That meant two people out of five would be missing during the busiest time. I hesitated, but as the towels were getting completely soaked and needed replacements, I had no choice but to ask Carmen. We ran to her car and she drove as fast as she could, exceeding the speed limit, and dropped me off at the ER. I asked her to go back to the deli as I went up to the registration window.

When the nurse saw the amount of blood coming from my nose, she completed the registration procedure as quickly as she could, handed me the form to sign, and walked me in to a treatment room. A few minutes later, the attending doctor came in and started working inside my nose. While he was administering to my problem, I was thinking about the deli. "I hope they'll be okay without me—the lines are probably all the way to the door," I mused. The doctor stabilized the bleeding and began repairing the veins inside my nose. Two hours later I was all fixed up. I thanked the doctor for a job well done and called the deli for someone to pick me up.

Everything returned to normal, and by the next day I had all but forgotten the incident. However, six months later I was diagnosed with colon cancer that revealed itself because of severe anemia. Now two years later I have learned that a person with anemia, which means low levels of iron in the blood, is subject to excessive bleeding from possible injury due to the difficulties the blood has coagulating. Had I known that after my incident, I might have suspected something was wrong with my health six months sooner, and it may have made a difference—something I will never know.

Dr. Day's tapes claimed that cancer doesn't just happen, that we cause it ourselves. I don't know if this is true, but I decided to examine what I could possibly have done to cause mine.

Five years earlier on July 4, 2000, Independence Day and also our wedding anniversary, we took a family holiday trip with our good friends Jackie and Joel's family to Lake Tahoe, Nevada. Among other activities, we visited beautiful Emerald Bay, which sits at the end of a very steep hill. On the way back I had great difficulties climbing the hill. As I was huffing and puffing, I recalled stepping on the scale before we left and discovering I weighed 185 pounds, which was the most I'd ever weighed. I totally forgot about the high elevation, which often makes it harder to breathe. Instead I decided I was way overweight and needed to go on a diet.

Several months before, I'd read a book, *Eat Right 4 Your Type* by Peter D'Adamo, that was given to me by a friend. Its basic theory was that most diets don't work because people with different blood types should have different diets. With a blood type of O positive, I needed to follow a diet based on meat, fish, and mostly fruits and vegetables—no pasta, no bread, and no white rice. According to the book, I should also avoid eating anything made from white flour that contained gluten and carbohydrates. I bought into this theory, and that very night during dinner I made the decision to start this diet and completely avoid eating bread. From that day on until my first surgery four-and-a-half years later, I followed this diet religiously, not even once cheating in any way. My daily breakfast consisted of a three-egg veggie omelet with tomatoes and green tea. Lunch and dinner always included meat or fish. No bread, no pasta, no white rice, but large quantities of green tea. I also ate large quantities of fruits and vegetables. The diet was successful and my weight went down to 160 pounds in six months. But in retrospect, I don't know how healthy it was to be eating three eggs every day along with large portions of red meat. Green tea was supposed to be healthy, but now I wasn't so sure of that either. Did this diet and the way I chose to practice it contribute in any way to my cancer? Of course there is no way to tell, but it may very well be.

Another possible cause could be my line of work. For sixteen years we ran a deli, and the food business can be very stressful at times. There are always deadlines to be met, catered lunches to be delivered at the same time and to several locations, and many other challenges. Stress has been known to cause harm and may well be a contributing factor for many health problems, which the National Cancer Institute says can include cancer. Some people know how to deal with it better than others. Unfortunately, I didn't know how to deal with it very well.

As I write these words, there is news about Tony Snow, President Bush's press secretary: his colon cancer returned two years after he had surgery to remove his colon. I couldn't help thinking about the level of stress that he was subject to in his line of work.

A third cause could be genetic. I was asked countless times if my parents or any of my close relatives had colon cancer, and as far as I knew, they didn't. But after my diagnosis, my younger brother had a colonoscopy done, and a number of polyps were found. A colonoscopy is a very good tool in the fight to prevent colon cancer, but unfortunately not enough people are undergoing this procedure. The recommendation by the American Gastroenterological Society is that every person over fifty should have one because this is the age group in which most new cases are diagnosed. It is worth emphasizing here the difference between prevention and early detection. A mammogram, for instance, is a tool used for early *detection* of breast cancer, and a large percentage of women over forty have the procedure. A colonoscopy is a tool that can actually *prevent* colon cancer by removing polyps that if left alone could become malignant tumors, yet a lot fewer people are taking advantage of it—which doesn't make a whole lot of sense. According to the American Cancer Society, if all adults fifty and older were screened for colon cancer, the death rate from this disease could be cut in half, saving approximately twenty-five thousand lives per year.

Here's an e-mail message I received from the American Cancer Society containing additional information:

> The following is the latest statistic from the American Cancer Society: "New cases: An estimated 108,070 cases of colon and 40,740 cases of rectal cancer are expected to occur in 2008. Colorectal cancer is the third most common cancer in both men and women. Colorectal cancer incidence rates have been decreasing for most of the last 2 decades (from 66.3 cases per 100,000 population in 1985 to 48.2 in 2004). The decline has been steeper in the most recent time period (2.3% per year from 1998–2004), partly due to an increase in screening, which can result in the detection and removal of colorectal polyps before they progress to cancer.

Deaths: An estimated 49,960 deaths from colon and rectum cancer are expected to occur in 2008, accounting for 9% of all cancer deaths.

Mortality rates from colorectal cancer have declined in both men and women over the past two decades with a steeper decline in the most recent time period (1.8% per year from 1985–2002 compared to 4.7% from 2002–2004). This decrease reflects declining incidence rates and improvements in early detection and treatment." (page 12)

There is also the environmental factor. We can't tell now what goes into our food or determine the quality of the air we breathe. We are causing so much damage to the environment that it's only reasonable to think there's a price to pay, although it's not yet easy to measure. Unfortunately, there's more unknown than known in the field of cancer research, but the advances made are measurable, and many lives are being saved.

My attempts to accurately pinpoint the cause of my cancer are doomed to fail. The only thing I know is that a colonoscopy, recommended at age fifty, could have allowed doctors to diagnose the polyps—small growths on the inner lining of the colon and rectum—and remove them, thus possibly preventing them from becoming cancerous. The lesson for all this may be that greater awareness and timely screening for colon cancer can make all the difference. According to Dr. F, no other type of cancer has a screening test that can prevent the disease—yet only 53 percent of the U.S. population is taking advantage of it.

More information on cancer statistics and patients' help can be found in the following Web sites:

http://www.cancer.org

http://www.seer.cancer.gov

http://www.monahancenter.org

http://www.aacr.org

http://www.aicr.org

http://www.acor.org

http://www.cancercare.org

http://www.cancerhopenetwork.org

http://www.cancer.gov

http://www.preventcancer.org

http://www.icare.org

http://www.uicc.org

http://www.nccra.org

http://www.ccalliance.org

http://www.colorectal-cancer.net

http://www.hereditarycc.org

http://www.acg.gi.org

http://www.gastro.org

http://www.fascrs.org

http://www.asge.org

http://www.ccfa.org

http://www.uoaa.org

19
A New Beginning

The last two years of my life were a time of crisis for my family and me, especially after my third surgery and subsequent chemotherapy. But as I gain strength on a daily basis, take longer walks on the trails of Palomares Hills where we live, and enjoy more time outdoors, I look at the last two years as a new beginning. I'm beginning to rediscover all the beautiful, small things that are easily overlooked in our busy lives: the nice warmth of the morning sun, the beautiful sounds of birds singing, the green carpet covering the hills after a rain, the wild rabbit crossing the path in front of me on the trail, the deer feeding on the tree outside our window, and all the other gifts given to us by nature. I'm gaining a greater appreciation for things usually taken for granted, and it brings immeasurable joy to my life.

I've also learned a few new things. I've learned that life is a precious gift. After confronting death, I now have a greater appreciation for all little pleasures in life. I'm very grateful for the second chance given to me to live life to its fullest. Things that used to make me upset or angry no longer have the same effect. I remember a book I read years ago, *Don't Sweat the Small Stuff ... and It's All Small Stuff* by Richard Carlson, and realize how true it is.

Another wonderful thing I started noticing again is the existence of the opposite sex, starting with my beautiful wife, Shoshi. During the time of my illness and recovery, my overwhelming thoughts were of survival and overcoming the challenges I faced. The department of sexuality in my brain was completely shut down. It was very exciting to rediscover these kinds of thoughts, which brings up the question: did my system survive the rerouting of the nerves and blood vessels inside my body organs? (After my first two surgeries, it took me about three weeks after being discharged to resume sexual activity.) The answer to this question was still unknown, and I eagerly awaited any evidence that the physical triggers were still connected. When Dr. W told me about the risks of losing the ability to achieve an erection, he could not tell me how many of his patients had suffered such a loss. He was sure that some of them did, but they weren't willing to report it.

Once I woke up in the middle of the night with an erection; this was the first time after the third surgery that this had happened, and it was very exciting news. However, when I woke up in the morning, I wasn't sure if it had really happened or if it was only a dream. But then the following night, the exact same thing happened. It took a little longer than before, but I was ready for sexual activity again.

As time went by, I became accustomed to the change in my personal hygiene. For example, I now had to wipe my butt from the front, which has some advantages, such as being able to better see what I am doing. And if absolutely necessary, it is possible to do this standing up—something I don't recommend to people whose colon is where nature put it. The ostomy bag has become a part of me, and I have learned to accept it. I look at it as a territory outside my body, as a sort of *colony*. And like some superpowers that used to dump their waste in the territory of their colonies, I do the same thing, but without having any guilty feelings about it.

As I was getting back in shape, I started running again for one or two miles and walking for five to six miles. Before too long I was able to walk around Lake Chabot again with my friend Motty—a nine-mile distance. I have not yet attempted a marathon, and it may very well never happen. But I feel healthy and fit, and I enjoy life. However, like every cancer patient, I have frequent tests just to make sure the cancer has not snuck back.

Helpful Hints

I thought it would be useful to include the following helpful hints to assist people in navigating an illness and getting the most out of a hospital stay. Here are a few things I have learned from my experience:

1. **Get Personally Involved in Your Treatment.** Get educated about your illness and the treatment your medical team is persuing by asking questions. Know all medications you're receiving, including dosage, frequency, and side effects. Be aware of different tests ordered for you and why. This will help you minimize mistakes and gain the respect of the medical staff.

2. **Be Nice.** Try not to be angry, rude, or demanding, and don't complain too much. The medical staff is there to help you get well, but there are many other patients just as important as you. If you become the person everybody is trying to avoid, it will set you back and delay your recovery.

3. **Get Family Support.** Having a supportive family is crucial for a speedy recovery. If you are lacking in this area, be extra friendly with your roommate(s) and their families, if they have one. Be extra friendly with all volunteers who come to visit and with all staff members. Maybe someone will "adopt" you for the duration of your hospital stay.

4. **Use Good Personal Hygiene.** Hospitals are not very clean places—they are full of germs. It's very important to wash your hands after bathroom visits and before eating as well as at every other opportunity. Take showers; if wet ones aren't possible, the dry ones are also good. Use the special moist towels the hospitals have. While in the hospital, we don't look or feel our best, so sometimes we're not motivated to take care of ourselves. This can be a mistake, as looking good usually also makes us feel good.

5. **Exercise.** Even in bed, exercise may be more important than ever. Just moving your ankles and hands can be helpful to your body, and so can lifting your legs or walking, if getting out of bed is an option. Doing whatever is possible can be very good for your blood flow and for your spirits.

6. **Get Fresh Air.** It's very likely viruses are around you, but as most hospitals don't give you the option of opening the windows, if possible, it is important to get outside. Walking is the best even if it means dragging the IV stand with you. But even if you're in a wheelchair, getting outdoors is worth the effort. It literally becomes a breath of fresh air.

7. **Have a Sense of Humor.** Laughter is a big contributor to our well-being. Having to be in the hospital is not very funny, but your ability to see the funny aspects of it can make your stay there feel shorter.

8. **Eat Nutritious Food.** You may think that hospital cafeterias serve only healthy foods, but that isn't so. I was very surprised to see how much junk food is on hospital menus. Consulting with a nutritionist and the doctors on the best foods for your specific situation can be very helpful.

9. **Listen to Music.** Today a wealth of gadgets can provide quality music for our listening enjoyment. I personally prefer classical music, but whatever your favorite, listening to music will make you feel better.

It worked for me, as when my son Avi brought me his MP3 player, I used it daily. Often volunteer musicians perform in hospitals. They are worth every effort, so try not to miss them.

10. **Have a Good Attitude.** My attitude toward my illness was that it was an obvious case of mistaken identity: this disease entered the wrong body by mistake, and it was my body's job to correct that error. When I say body, I also mean mind. The mind is a very powerful part of the body. I used to visualize the cancer exiting my body and apologizing to me for having the wrong address.

11. **Get Out of There ASAP.** Hospitals are necessary places to regain our good health with the help of caring professionals; they are not good places for vacationing. My goal was to get strong enough that I could continue my recovery at home. Your recovery time will be much faster when you are surrounded by loving family, friends, and acquaintances.

** ** ** ** ** **

Cancer gave me the opportunity to step out of my comfort zone and write, something I'd never tried before. I've discovered that although very difficult, sharing my story and expressing my feelings has a side benefit of a healing effect. And if my story can help others facing similar challenges—as I was helped and inspired by reading Brenda Elsagher's in her book, *If the Battle Is Over, Why am I Still in Uniform?*—this will be my greatest reward.

When I was a new immigrant to this country in the early 1980s, I was faced with enormous challenges—economical, social, and marital. I read a book by Robert H. Schuller, *Tough Times Never Last, but Tough People Do.* This book was instrumental in getting me through the difficult times. Little did I know then that more challenges would be coming my way, and remembering this book was a big help. The passage of time helps us forget even the worst of times. Even my more recent health challenges started fading from my memory as soon as I regained my health. Our brains have the capacity to move on, so if we can just tough it out during the hard times, better times are sure to follow.

Acknowledgments

I would like to thank all the people who stood shoulder to shoulder with me in my battles. First, I thank my super family: my wife, Shoshi, who checked herself into the hospital with me and provided immeasurable love, support, and care throughout my hospital stay and my subsequent follow-ups and chemo treatments; and my children, Avi, Yaniv, and Orit, also for their love and support as well as their help with all the research and running our business in our absence. Second, I thank Dr. Welton, Dr. Fisher, Dr. Lowe, and all the staff at Stanford Hospital for saving my life. A special thank you goes to Dr. Shlomo Hellerstein and his wonderful wife, Aviva. Dr. Hellerstein took a personal interest in my recovery and provided on-demand advice and counsel, expecting nothing in return from the first time I was diagnosed until this day. Thank you to Margaret Love, Dr. Fischer's assistant, for organizing and running the support group that played an important role in my healing process. I would also like to thank Denise Hodges for her skillful editing and for her patience and commitment. It was a joy working with her on this project.

Useful Definitions

Term	Definition
Adenocarcinoma	Cancer that develops in cells lining glandular types of internal organs
Adjuvant chemotherapy	Drugs or hormones given after surgery in an effort to prevent the cancer from coming back
Alopecia	Hair loss
Anemia	Having too few red blood cells
Antiemetic	Medication to prevent nausea and vomiting
Benign	Not cancerous
Blood cell count	The number of red and white blood cells and platelets in a sample of blood. A complete blood count is called a *CBC*.
Bone marrow	The inner tissue of bones where blood cells are made
Cancer	Term for many diseases in which cells grow out of control
Catheter	Thin, flexible tube through which fluids leave or enter the body
CBC	Complete blood cell count (see *blood cell count*, above)
CEA	Carcinoembryonic antigen, a blood test used to mark the stage and extent of a cancer

Term	Definition
Central venous catheter	Special thin and flexible tube placed in a large vein that remains there for as long as needed to deliver and withdraw fluids
Chemotherapy	The use of drugs to treat cancer
Clinical trials	Studies that test new drugs on human volunteers in order to discover new and better treatments for cancer and other diseases
Colon	The part of the large intestine that is connected to the rectum
Colonoscopy	The examination of the colon using a flexible, lighted instrument called a colonoscope
Colostomy	Surgical procedure that creates an opening in the abdomen for a part of the large intestine; replaces the rectum
Combination chemotherapy	The use of more than one drug to treat cancer
CT scan	Computed tomography; an imaging method that uses X-rays to create cross-sectional pictures of the body
Diuretic	Substance that depletes water and salt from the body
ECG	Electrocardiogram; a test that records the electrical activity of the heart
ER	Emergency room
GI	Gastrointestinal; the digestive tract

Term	Definition
Hemicolectomy	Procedure in which a portion of the large bowel is removed due to the presence of cancer. This may involve either the left or right part of the bowel.
Hormones	Substances produced by the endocrine glands that are released directly into the bloodstream
Infusion	Intravenous delivery of a drug or fluids
Injection	Use of a syringe and needle to deliver fluids or drugs into the body
IV	Intravenous; into a vein
Laparotomy	Diagnostic procedure used to assess disease in the abdomen. One of the more frequent reasons for a laparotomy is to determine the extent to which a cancer has spread.
Lymph nodes	Glands that trap foreign particles and help the body fight viruses, bacteria, and disease
Malignant	Cancerous
Normal range	Term used to describe the optimal, desired range for test results. A result out of this normal range is sometimes a signal that further investigation is needed.
Oncologist	Physician who specializes in cancer
Ostomy	Surgical opening created for the elimination of bodily waste

Term	Definition
Peripheral neuropathy	Condition of the nervous system that causes numbness or tingling, usually of the hands and feet; a side effect of chemotherapy.
PET scan	Positron emission tomography scan; a diagnostic examination that uses nuclear medicine medical imaging techniques to produce three-dimensional images used to evaluate cancer and other diseases
Platelets	Blood cells that stop bleeding
Port	Catheter surgically placed under the skin to deliver and withdraw fluids instead of an IV tube.
Radiation therapy	High-energy rays used to treat cancer
Radiologist	Physician who specializes in radiology, the field of diagnosis and treatment of disease with the help of radiation
RBCs	Red blood cells, which supply oxygen to all tissues in the body
Remission	The partial or complete disappearance of cancer
Staging system	A standardized classification scheme explaining the extent of a cancer that allows physicians to quickly and accurately describe a patient's cancer using a universal language that all specialists can understand

Term	Definition
Stoma	Surgically created opening in the abdomen to replace the rectum
Stoma nurse	Nurse specializing in the care of patients with a stoma wound
Tumor	An uncontrolled growth of cells or tissues that may be benign or malignant
UOAA	United Ostomy Association of America
WBCs	White blood cells, which fight infection

www.ingramcontent.com/pod-product-compliance
Lightning Source LLC
Chambersburg PA
CBHW051432280526
45785CB00003B/1258

www.ingramcontent.com/pod-product-compliance
Lightning Source LLC
Chambersburg PA
CBHW051434280526
45785CB00003B/1283